New COVID-19 Variants - Diagnosis and Management in the Post-Pandemic Era

Edited by Ozgur Karcioglu

Published in London, United Kingdom

New COVID-19 Variants - Diagnosis and Management in the Post-Pandemic Era
http://dx.doi.org/10.5772/intechopen.111256
Edited by Ozgur Karcioglu

Contributors
Abad Ali Nadeem, Amina Nazir, Amit Kumar Tripathi, Ana Sánchez Tlapalcoyoatl, Asanda Mayeye, Bakhtawar Bukhari, Charles Shey Wiysonge, Duduzile Ndwandwe, Efraín Navarro-Olivos, Fatima Akram, Francisco Javier Magos-Vázquez, Fuad Pašić, Gabriela González Cannata, Gilberto Flores-Vargas, Guadalupe Irazú Morales-Reyes, Ishrat Perveen, Jessica Paola Plascencia-Roldán, Kajal Singh, Khushi Gandhi, Lahcen Belyamani, Liping Li, Longlong Zuo, Luis Ulises Pérez-Arenas, Lulu Li, María de Jesús Gallardo-Luna, Mouna Ouadghiri, Muhammad Farooq, Musawenkosi Ndlovu, Naaz Abbas, Nancy Singh, Ndivhuwo Muvhulawa, Nicolás Padilla-Raygoza, Nomahlubi Luphondo, Peijun Zuo, Phiwayinkosi V. Dludla, Quratulain Syed, Rachid El Jaoudi, Ramsha Essa, Richa Das, Rosa María Romero Castro, Saba Sabahat, Safae El Mazouri, Samia Nawab, Sana Riaz, Sania Mazhar, Sara Louati, Shaista Nawaz, Shreni Agrawal, Syed Hussain Imam Abidi, Tarik Aanniz, Xiaonan Zhao, Yasar Saleem, Yeter Eylül Bayram, Yibao Chen, Yonela Ntamo, Yuqing Liu, Zhihong Li

First published in London, United Kingdom, 2024 by IntechOpen
IntechOpen is the global imprint of INTECHOPEN LIMITED, registered in England and Wales, registration number: 11086078, 167-169 Great Portland Street, London, W1W 5PF, United Kingdom

British Library Cataloguing-in-Publication Data
A catalogue record for this book is available from the British Library

Additional hard and PDF copies can be obtained from orders@intechopen.com

New COVID-19 Variants - Diagnosis and Management in the Post-Pandemic Era
Edited by Ozgur Karcioglu
p. cm.
Print ISBN 978-0-85466-173-2
Online ISBN 978-0-85466-172-5
eBook (PDF) ISBN 978-0-85466-174-9

For EU product safety concerns:
IN TECH d.o.o., Prolaz Marije Krucifikse Kozulić 3, 51000 Rijeka, Croatia,
info@intechopen.com or visit our website at intechopen.com.

Meet the editor

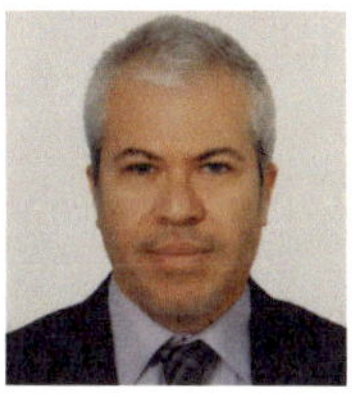

Dr. Ozgur Karcioglu graduated from his residency at the Department of Emergency Medicine, Dokuz Eylul University, Turkey, in 1998. He completed a fellowship in international emergency medicine at Penn State University, USA, in 2005. He is currently the chair and residency director of the Department of Emergency Medicine, Istanbul-Taksim Education and Research Hospital. He is a founder of the Emergency Medical Association of Turkey. He is the editor and author of numerous books. His research interests include resuscitation, advanced life support, pain management, airway emergencies, geriatrics, disaster medicine, trauma, toxicology, and COVID-19.

Contents

Preface **IX**

Section 1
Diagnostic and Descriptive Characteristics of COVID-19 Variants **1**

Chapter 1 **3**
Multisystem Inflammatory Syndrome in Adult (MIS-A)
by Yeter Eylül Bayram

Chapter 2 **19**
Omicron: A SARS-CoV-2 Variant
by Khushi Gandhi

Chapter 3 **39**
Production and Formation of SARS-CoV-2 Variants
by Ishrat Perveen, Bakhtawar Bukhari, Naaz Abbas, Sania Mazhar, Yasar Saleem, Shaista Nawaz, Samia Nawab, Quratulain Syed, Syed Hussain Imam Abidi, Sana Riaz, Ramsha Essa, Abad Ali Nadeem, Muhammad Farooq, Fatima Akram and Saba Sabahat

Chapter 4 **55**
Understanding the Omicron Variant in the COVID-19 Pandemic
by Safae El Mazouri, Tarik Aanniz, Sara Louati, Lahcen Belyamani, Rachid El Jaoudi and Mouna Ouadghiri

Chapter 5 **73**
Virulence and Infectivity Were Associated with Different Fragments in the Delta Subtype of SARS-CoV-2
by Peijun Zuo, Longlong Zuo, Zhihong Li and Liping Li

Chapter 6 **91**
Unraveling the Significance of Phage-Derived Enzymes for Treating Secondary Bacterial Infections among COVID-19 Patients
by Amina Nazir, Lulu Li, Xiaonan Zhao, Yuqing Liu and Yibao Chen

Chapter 7 **111**
SARS-CoV-2 (COVID-19) Variants in Mexico
by Luis Ulises Pérez-Arenas, Jessica Paola Plascencia-Roldán, Guadalupe Irazú Morales-Reyes, Gilberto Flores-Vargas, María de Jesús Gallardo-Luna, Efraín Navarro-Olivos, Francisco Javier Magos-Vázquez and Nicolás Padilla-Raygoza

Section 2
Specific Organ Effects and Treatment Principles **127**

Chapter 8 **129**
Spontaneous Hemorrhage in COVID 19 Patients
by Fuad Pašić

Chapter 9 **143**
Posterior Segment Ocular Findings in Critically Ill Patients with COVID
by Rosa María Romero Castro, Gabriela González Cannata and Ana Sánchez Tlapalcoyoatl

Chapter 10 **155**
Managing COVID-19 Variants: Mapping Data from the International Clinical Trials Registry Platform
by Duduzile Ndwandwe, Musawenkosi Ndlovu, Asanda Mayeye, Nomahlubi Luphondo, Ndivhuwo Muvhulawa, Yonela Ntamo, Phiwayinkosi V. Dludla and Charles Shey Wiysonge

Chapter 11 **173**
Impact of New COVID-19 Variant on Stroke, Thrombosis and Neurological Impairment
by Richa Das, Shreni Agrawal, Nancy Singh, Kajal Singh and Amit Kumar Tripathi

Preface

COVID-19 is a major cause of preventable deaths throughout the world. Although four years have passed since the beginning of the COVID-19 pandemic, COVID-19 is not over. According to data from the World Health Organization (WHO) and the Centers for Disease Control (CDC), there were more than 700 million confirmed cases and almost 7 million deaths due to COVID worldwide as of January 20, 2024, which is a mortality rate of 1%. COVID-19 killed around 100,000 Americans in 2023. That is much more than what would be considered a "bad" flu year. The elderly account for most deaths and ICU hospitalizations throughout the world. It is postulated that the number of COVID-19 cases may increase in the coming period due to new variants. It is concerning that the virus may evade vaccine and disease-associated immunity. Long COVID affects nearly every tissue of the human body, including the neurocognitive and cardiovascular systems.

COVID-19 symptoms vary depending on the specific variant and may include sore throat, cough, congestion, runny nose, headache, muscle/body aches, fatigue, sneezing, fever/chills, nausea/vomiting, loss of taste/smell, diarrhea, and shortness of breath. It is not a surprise that the number of cases increases as flu season arrives and the weather gets colder. The increases in COVID-19 infections starting from 2023 are also related to other subjective factors, such as declining immunity, newly emerging variants, and delay in access to updated booster vaccines.

COVID-19 poses the greatest threat to the elderly, those with compromised immune systems, pregnant women, or people with certain health conditions such as diabetes, obesity, and chronic lung diseases. People with COVID-19 are infectious starting from about two days before developing symptoms (in the presymptomatic period) or the date of a positive test. They continue to spread the virus to other people for up to 10 days after developing symptoms or, if asymptomatic, until 10 days after the date of a positive test. This supports that vaccines are more effective than masks for protection.

It is vital to take the necessary precautions to protect society, especially elderly and chronic patients, from both COVID-19 and other infectious diseases, learning from the mistakes made earlier in the pandemic. Measures should include combating vaccine hesitancy, with the participation of society. A CDC study found that surgical masks used in indoor public settings reduce the likelihood of contracting the coronavirus by 66%. Thus, we should wear masks to protect ourselves and our loved ones in crowded and poorly ventilated-places. Wearing a high-quality mask as well as getting vaccinated and boosted will largely prevent hospitalizations and deaths.

Vaccination is our most important protection. Globally, 13.53 billion doses have been administered, and 9614 are now administered each day. Recorded deaths are clearly approaching zero in groups with effective vaccination. The CDC recommends updated COVID-19 booster vaccines for everyone 6 months and older. Although there is insufficient efficacy data for children under the age of 12, the decision to update the booster for children was made accordingly. Updated vaccines from Moderna, Pfizer, and Novavax have been available since summer 2023. Updating with bivalent vaccines has been recommended in recent years for people older than 65 years. Pneumonia vaccines for elderly patients and influenza vaccines for all risk groups should also be brought back to the agenda. Especially in developing countries, the state can have difficulties in prioritizing vaccination and other measures for public health. Science and open-mindedness will save the planet, as long as the state and the public act in unison to see that the next generations remain healthy.

Ozgur Karcioglu
Department of Emergency Medicine,
Taksim Training and Research Hospital,
University of Health Sciences,
Istanbul, Turkey

Section 1

Diagnostic and Descriptive Characteristics of COVID-19 Variants

Chapter 1

Multisystem Inflammatory Syndrome in Adult (MIS-A)

Yeter Eylül Bayram

Abstract

Multisystem Inflammatory Syndrome (MIS) is a severe medical condition that can develop following a COVID-19 infection. It is characterized by widespread tissue inflammation, affecting various organs such as the heart, lungs, kidneys, brain, skin, eyes, and gastrointestinal system. A new medical condition emerged in children during the early stages of the COVID-19 pandemic. This condition necessitated intensive care due to symptoms like fever, abdominal pain, heart failure, and shock, which could lead to fatal outcomes. This condition bore some similarities to Kawasaki disease and was named 'Multisystemic Inflammatory Syndrome in Children (MIS-C)' by the Centers for Disease Control and Prevention (CDC) in April 2020. Subsequently, similar clinical conditions were reported in adults in June 2020, and this condition in adults was defined as 'MIS-A.' MIS-A primarily affects individuals aged 21 and older. It is characterized by persistent fever, multi-organ involvement, elevated markers of systemic inflammation, a history of exposure to SARS-CoV-2, and the absence of an alternative diagnosis. Early diagnosis of MIS-A is crucial, as a delayed diagnosis can be life-threatening.

Keywords: COVID-19, adults, SARS-CoV-2, multisystem inflammatory syndrome, diagnose, treatment

1. Introduction

In December 2019, an outbreak of pneumonia with an unidentified cause emerged in Wuhan, China [1]. Subsequently, it was determined that a novel coronavirus was responsible for the disease, leading to its designation as Severe Acute Respiratory Syndrome Coronavirus 2 (SARS-CoV-2). This disease became known as Coronavirus Disease 2019 (COVID-19). The virus swiftly spread globally, prompting the World Health Organization (WHO) to declare it a global pandemic on March 11, 2020 [2].

SARS-CoV-2 is an enveloped, single-stranded positive RNA virus belonging to the beta coronavirus family. Its spike (S) glycoprotein binds to angiotensin-converting enzyme 2 (ACE2), a transmembrane protein highly expressed in vascular endothelial cells within the lungs and other organs. This interaction facilitates the virus's entry into host cells, triggering an immune response that includes the production of pro-inflammatory cytokines [3]. This immune response can sometimes lead to severe conditions such as acute respiratory distress syndrome (ARDS), multi-organ failure, and even death in infected individuals [4].

COVID-19 presents with a range of symptoms, varying from asymptomatic or mild to severe. Common symptoms include dry cough, sore throat, fever, shortness of breath, fatigue, sputum production, dyspnea, conjunctivitis, myalgia, and loss of taste or smell [5]. The severity of the disease is categorized as mild, moderate, severe, or critical. COVID-19 progresses through three stages: early infection with the viral invasion of host cells, a pulmonary phase characterized by lung tissue damage due to immune activation and proinflammatory cascades, and the most dangerous phase, the inflammatory cell overactivation period known as the cytokine storm [6]. This phase can result in respiratory distress, oxygen desaturation, respiratory failure, and an increased risk of venous thromboembolism [7].

In children, COVID-19 generally follows a milder course compared to adults, and many children may remain asymptomatic [8]. However, in April 2020, a new condition characterized by severe inflammation, like Kawasaki disease and toxic shock syndrome, was observed in previously healthy children who had recently been infected with SARS-CoV-2 [9]. Affected children displayed symptoms such as high fever, abdominal pain, hypotension, myocardial dysfunction, multi-organ failure, and the need for intensive care. Epidemiological analysis revealed a delay of several weeks between the peak of COVID-19 cases in the community and the highest number of MIS-C cases. This suggests a potential link to post-infection immune responses [10].

The first reports of these cases in Europe came from the UK, and this new condition was temporarily named Pediatric Inflammatory Multisystem Syndrome temporally associated with SARS-CoV-2 (PIMS-TS) by the Royal College of Pediatrics and Child Health (RCPCH). Subsequently, similar case reports emerged from the United States, leading to the CDC and WHO defining it as Multisystem Inflammatory Syndrome in Children (MIS-C) in April 2020 [11].

As the COVID-19 pandemic continued, similar clinical findings were reported in adults who had previously been infected with SARS-CoV-2. In June 2020, this condition seen in adults was defined as MIS-A [12, 13].

2. MIS-A pathophysiology

MIS-A is a rare complication of COVID-19, and its pathophysiology is not yet fully understood, but it can be potentially life-threatening. Clinically, the disease most commonly manifests itself 2–6 weeks after infection, especially affecting young and middle-aged patients [14]. The clinical course of the disease is highly variable, with fever being the most important clinical sign and the most observed symptom. Additionally, widespread organ involvement and signs of shock can occur due to systemic inflammation [15].

The exact pathophysiology of MIS-A remains uncertain, but it is suggested to result from a delayed and irregular immune response that occurs weeks after recovery from COVID-19 infection. In most cases of SARS-CoV-2 infection, there is an inflammatory immune response that activates both the innate and acquired immune systems. However, during the recovery period, an irregular immune response, possibly contributed to by macrophage activation, can lead to hyperinflammation. This results in the reactivation of both the innate and acquired immune systems, involving B cells and T cells, along with high levels of proinflammatory production. Cytokines and antibodies play a role in this process. These inflammatory cytokines lead to a multisystem inflammatory response and contribute to the development of MIS-A [16, 17].

The exact cause of this irregular immune response that develops after recovering from COVID-19 infection is not known, but it is believed to be related to persistent viral antigens and autoantibodies [18].

3. Clinical symptoms of MIS-A

In MIS-A, there is a severe systemic inflammatory response accompanied by multi-organ dysfunction, including the heart, lungs, kidneys, brain, skin, eyes, or gastrointestinal system, along with elevated proinflammatory markers. Symptoms can often appear 2–6 weeks after SARS-CoV-2 virus infection. The most common symptom and clinical finding in MIS-A patients is fever. Unlike most infectious diseases, MIS-A patients typically have persistent and prolonged fever. In addition to fever, clinical symptoms observed in MIS-A can include abdominal pain, vomiting, diarrhea, various skin lesions, non-purulent conjunctivitis (bloodshot eyes), shortness of breath, myalgia (muscle pain), headache, encephalopathy, newly developed epileptic seizures, dizziness, and clinical symptoms of hypotension and shock. In the case of the series, it has been reported that 100% of patients had a fever (fever being a prerequisite for diagnosis), and skin rash was seen in 57.8% of cases. Diarrhea (51.6%) and abdominal pain (40.6%) were also noted as the most common gastrointestinal symptoms in MIS-A [14, 15, 17].

Characteristics of organ involvement in MIS-A include:

Multi-Organ Involvement: MIS-A can affect various organs, including the heart, lungs, kidneys, gastrointestinal system, and skin. Patients may experience symptoms related to dysfunction in these organs, such as chest pain, shortness of breath, abdominal pain, diarrhea, and skin rashes [18].

Heart: Cardiac involvement is common in MIS-A and is among the main causes of mortality and morbidity. The most common cardiac abnormalities observed include myocarditis (inflammation of the heart muscle), pericarditis (inflammation of the lining around the heart), pericardial effusion, coronary artery dilatation or aneurysm, echocardiographic findings indicating left or right ventricular dysfunction, elevated levels of troponin and BNP (B-type Natriuretic Peptide), various arrhythmic electrocardiogram abnormalities such as second and third-degree atrioventricular (A-V) block, ventricular tachycardia, along with hypotension or cardiogenic shock. Patients may also present with chest pain, and symptoms related to hypotension or cardiac shock can be observed. Additionally, in previously reported cases, cardiac involvement in MIS-A has been observed to be reversible, with improved heart function seen in follow-up assessments [17, 19].

Skin: The skin is one of the most affected organs in MIS-A. Skin rashes are typically widespread and may have a maculopapular and/or polymorphic character. Patients may experience non-exudative conjunctivitis, periorbital edema, mucositis, subcutaneous edema, palmar erythema, and petechial rashes. Vesicular rashes are not expected in the MIS-A [17, 18, 20].

Gastrointestinal system: Gastrointestinal symptoms in MIS-A can include abdominal pain, vomiting, or diarrhea. In the reported case series, diarrhea (51.6%) and abdominal pain (40.6%) were noted as the most common gastrointestinal symptoms. While gastrointestinal symptoms tend to be dominant in MIS-C patients, traditional Kawasaki disease (KD) symptoms like vomiting and diarrhea are rare [18, 21].

Brain: Neurological symptoms and signs may include newly developed headaches, encephalopathy, meningeal signs, epileptic seizures, or peripheral neuropathy. Newly developed Guillain-Barré syndrome is also considered one of the peripheral neurological findings in the MIS-A [16, 17]. These features, along with multi-organ dysfunction and elevated proinflammatory markers, contribute to the serious systemic inflammatory response seen in MIS-A.

It's important to note that the observed findings in MIS-A are not specific and can also occur in other infectious diseases and inflammatory conditions. The heterogeneity of clinical symptoms in MIS-A can make diagnosis challenging for clinicians. In a patient suspected of having a multisystemic inflammatory disease with persistent high fever and a history of exposure to the SARS-CoV-2 virus, advanced investigations are recommended if at least two of the listed findings are present to establish the diagnosis of MIS-A [15, 17].

It's clear from the various studies and reports you have mentioned that MIS-A (Multisystem Inflammatory Syndrome in Adults) is a complex and serious condition associated with previous COVID-19 infection. Here are some key findings from the literature:

1. CDC report (2020):

    - In 2020, the CDC (Centers for Disease Control and Prevention) reported 27 cases that met the criteria for MIS-A.

    - The patients' ages ranged from 21 to 50 years.

    - Common symptoms included fever, gastrointestinal symptoms, and ground-glass images in some cases.

    - All patients showed increased inflammatory markers, cardiac involvement, and positive PCR or antibody tests indicating prior COVID-19 infection.

    - Nine patients had no underlying medical conditions, while others had comorbidities like obesity, diabetes mellitus type 2, hypertension, and obstructive sleep apnea.

    - Some patients had negative PCR but positive antibody tests.

    - Most patients survived, but many required intensive care [6].

2. Belay et al. study:

    - The median age of 35 years in their case series.

    - 65% of the patients were male.

    - Most patients had a preceding COVID-19-like illness about a month before MIS-A onset [22].

3. Kunal S et al. study:

    - The review included 79 cases from 53 articles.

    - Most patients were male (73.4%) with a mean age of 31.67 years.

- Fever was the most common symptom, followed by skin rash.
- The cardiovascular system was most frequently involved, followed by the gastrointestinal system and mucocutaneous.
- Decreased left ventricular ejection fraction was observed in many patients.
- The mean time from symptom onset to hospital admission was about 5.84 days.
- Comorbidities like hypertension and obesity were common.
- The mean time to symptom onset before MIS-A in patients with previous COVID-19 infection was around 31.61 days [18].

4. Patel et al. review:

- A review of 221 MIS-A patients worldwide.
- MIS-A typically develops about 4 weeks after acute COVID-19 infection.
- The mean age was 21 years, with 70% being male, and 58% had no other comorbidities.
- Common symptoms included fever, hypotension, cardiac dysfunction, dyspnea, and diarrhea.
- Many patients required intensive care and respiratory support.
- The mortality rate was 7% [15].

These findings collectively highlight the diverse clinical presentations and outcomes associated with MIS-A, emphasizing the importance of timely recognition and management of this condition, especially in individuals with a recent history of COVID-19. Further research is needed to better understand the underlying mechanisms and improve clinical management strategies [14].

4. Laboratory findings

The laboratory findings associated with MIS-A (Multisystem Inflammatory Syndrome in Adults) typically reveal a significant increase in various inflammatory markers. Here are some key laboratory findings mentioned in the provided information:

1. Inflammatory markers:

- C-reactive protein (CRP): Elevated in most cases.
- Ferritin: Elevated.
- Interleukin 6 (IL-6): Elevated.

- Erythrocyte Sedimentation Rate: Elevated.
- Procalcitonin (PCT): Elevated.
- Fibrinogen: Elevated.
- D-dimer: Elevated.
- Lactate Dehydrogenase (LDH): Elevated.
- Lymphopenia: Reduced lymphocyte count.
- Thrombocytopenia: Reduced platelet count [17, 18].

2. Cardiac evaluation:

- Electrocardiogram (ECG): Recommended for cardiac assessment.
- Cardiac enzymes:
  - Troponin: Elevated in many cases.
  - B-type Natriuretic Peptide (BNP) /N-terminal-prohormone of brain Natriuretic Peptide (NT-pro BNP): Elevated.
- Echocardiography (ECHO): Recommended for assessing cardiac function.
- Left Ventricular Ejection Fraction (LVEF): Reduced in a significant percentage of cases (LVEF<50%).
- Right Ventricular Dysfunction: Present in some cases.
- Cardiac Magnetic Resonance (CMR): Myocardial edema and pericardial effusion were observed in some cases [15, 18].

3. SARS-CoV-2 testing:

- RT-PCR: Positive in some patients.
- Serology: Positive in most patients [17, 23].

These findings emphasize the importance of conducting thorough laboratory assessments and cardiac evaluations when diagnosing and managing MIS-A. Elevated inflammatory markers, cardiac involvement, and history of COVID-19 infection (PCR or antibody positivity) are common features in MIS-A patients. Additionally, coagulopathy and abnormalities in inflammatory parameters are frequently observed, underlining the systemic nature of this condition. Early diagnosis and appropriate management are crucial for improving patient outcomes [6, 23].

5. Case definition

The MIS-A (Multisystem Inflammatory Syndrome in Adults) case definition developed by the CDC (Centers for Disease Control and Prevention) in 2021 outlines the criteria that a patient must meet to be diagnosed with MIS-A. To be classified as a MIS-A case, a patient must:

1. Be 21 years of age or older.

2. Have an illness that resulted in hospitalization for 24 hours or longer or led to death.

3. Meet the following clinical and laboratory criteria, with alternative diagnoses ruled out:

    - Experience subjective fever lasting for ≥24 hours or documented fever (≥ 38.0°C) within the first 3 days before or after hospitalization. If we assume the admission date as day 0, these criteria must be met by the end of the third day.

    - Exhibit at least three of the following clinical criteria, with at least one being a primary clinical criterion:

- Primary clinical criteria:

    a. Severe cardiac illness, including myocarditis, pericarditis, coronary artery dilatation/aneurysm, or new-onset right or left ventricular dysfunction (LVEF<50%), 2nd/3rd-degree atrioventricular (A-V) block, or ventricular tachycardia (cardiac arrest alone does not meet this criterion).

    b. Rash AND non-purulent conjunctivitis.

- Secondary clinical criteria:

    a. New-onset neurologic signs and symptoms, including encephalopathy in a patient without prior cognitive impairment, seizures, meningeal signs, or peripheral neuropathy (including Guillain-Barré syndrome).

    b. Shock or hypotension not explained by medical therapy (e.g., sedation, renal replacement therapy).

    c. Abdominal pain, vomiting, or diarrhea.

    d. Thrombocytopenia (platelet count <150,000/microliter).

4. Provide laboratory evidence of inflammation AND SARS-CoV-2 infection, which includes:

    - Elevated levels of at least two of the following: C-reactive protein (CRP), ferritin, IL-6, erythrocyte sedimentation rate, and procalcitonin (PCT).

- A positive SARS-CoV-2 test result for current or recent infection by RT-PCR (reverse transcription-polymerase chain reaction), serology, or antigen detection [24].

This case definition helps healthcare professionals identify and diagnose MIS-A in adults while excluding other potential diagnoses. It focuses on clinical symptoms, laboratory markers, and the presence of SARS-CoV-2 infection to establish the MIS-A diagnosis [16].

6. Differential diagnosis

MIS-A can share many clinical features with other diseases such as Kawasaki Disease (KD), Toxic Shock Syndrome (TSS), Macrophage Activation Syndrome (MAS), and septic shock. Therefore, among adult patients who exhibit unexplained shock, heart failure, and/or gastrointestinal symptoms, MIS-A should be considered for diagnosis, even if there is no confirmed history of COVID-19 [23, 25].

Especially in children, MIS-C (Multisystem Inflammatory Syndrome in Children) shares similarities with Kawasaki Disease [8].

7. Kawasaki disease

Kawasaki disease is a condition that typically affects children under the age of 5 and is characterized by clinical symptoms such as fever, rash, conjunctivitis, swelling of the hands and feet, swollen neck lymph nodes, and inflammation of the mouth, lips, and throat.

According to the CDC, the diagnostic criteria for Kawasaki disease include:

1. Rash

2. Cervical lymph node enlargement (at least 1.5 cm in diameter)

3. Conjunctival inflammation in both eyes

4. Changes in oral mucosa

5. Changes in peripheral extremities

The diagnosis of Kawasaki disease is made when at least four of these five criteria are present along with fever. Two or three of the five main features, along with fever, are referred to as "incomplete Kawasaki [26].

Although Kawasaki Disease is generally a self-limiting condition, serious complications such as coronary artery aneurysms, myocardial dysfunction, and thrombotic events may develop in some children. Therefore, children diagnosed with Kawasaki Disease are typically treated with standard methods such as intravenous immunoglobulin and aspirin [27].

8. Differences between KD and MIS-C

When we compare Kawasaki disease (KD), which affects children and is extremely rare in adults, with MIS-C, we find several differences. In MIS-C cases, the average age is higher (with average ages of 8.5 for MIS-C and 3 for KD). While both diseases share fever as a common symptom and sign, there are variations in other aspects [6]:

1. Skin Rash: Skin rashes are slightly more common in MIS-C compared to KD.

2. Gastrointestinal Symptoms: Gastrointestinal symptoms such as vomiting, abdominal pain, and diarrhea tend to be more dominant in MIS-C, whereas, in traditional KD, gastrointestinal involvement is rare.

3. Inflammatory Markers: MIS-C is associated with higher levels of inflammatory markers such as C-reactive protein (CRP), ferritin, and D-dimer. Additionally, MIS-C patients often exhibit more lymphopenia and thrombocytopenia.

4. Cardiac Involvement: MIS-C typically has more severe cardiac involvement. High troponin levels, BNP (B-type natriuretic peptide), and EKG (electrocardiogram) changes are more common in MIS-C. Hypotension and shock are also more frequent in MIS-C.

5. Myocardial Edema: In KD, myocardial edema is often observed without ischemia, whereas MIS-C can lead to more severe myocardial involvement.

6. Mortality Rate: The mortality rate for MIS-C is higher (around 2%) compared to KD (around 0.17%) [6].

9. Differences between MIS-A and MIS-C

These distinctions are important for healthcare professionals when evaluating and diagnosing children with these conditions to ensure appropriate management and care. MIS-C and MIS-A are similar in many ways. However, MIS-C is more common than MIS-A. Accompanying comorbidities, the severity of cardiac dysfunction, incidence of thrombosis, shock, and mortality rate higher in MIS-A (**Table 1**) [6, 17].

We had mentioned earlier that MIS-A shares various clinical features with other diseases such as sepsis, septic shock, or toxic shock syndrome [14, 25]. This makes diagnosis difficult and can lead to delayed or missed appropriate treatment. A comprehensive history, physical examination, and laboratory investigation are necessary [14, 15]. Exposure to water sources and animals should be questioned to assess the risk of these diseases. Bacterial infections (such as staphylococcus, streptococcus, leptospirosis, and rickettsia) can cause toxic shock syndrome or septic shock. Therefore, these should also be considered in the differential diagnosis. Among common viral infections, viruses that can cause multi-system organ involvement, such as enteroviruses, adenoviruses, parvovirus, rotavirus, and Epstein-Barr

Phenotype	MIS-A	MIS-C
Prevalence	Less common	More Common
Myocarditis	54%	29%
Cardiac dysfunction	30%	15%
Arterial thrombosis, pulmonary embolism, and/or deep venous thrombosis	5%	1%
Dermatologic findings	46%	76%
Hospital stays	~8 days	~5 days
Ventilation	25%	9%
Sex	70% male	60% male
Mortality	7%	1%

Summarizing differences between MIS-A and MIS-C [6].
MIS-A shares various clinical features with other diseases such as sepsis, septic shock, or toxic shock syndrome, making its diagnosis challenging and potentially leading to delayed or missed appropriate treatment [17]. Bacterial sepsis is a significant concern in patients presenting with fever, shock, and elevated inflammatory markers. To differentiate MIS-A from bacterial sepsis, blood cultures should be obtained from all patients with suspected serious MIS-A, and empirical antibiotics should be administered while awaiting culture results. Some clinical characteristics may aid in distinguishing MIS-A from bacterial sepsis. For instance, cardiac involvement, especially coronary artery involvement, is rare in bacterial sepsis. Additionally, microbiological tests (SARS-CoV-2 antigen/antibody/RT-PCR tests, bacterial cultures) are necessary for differentiation [14, 17].

Table 1.
Differences between MIS-A and MIS-C.

virus (EBV), should be particularly kept in mind during differential diagnosis. Additionally, drug-induced hypersensitivity syndrome (DIHS) and macrophage activation syndrome (MAS), which can lead to a similar clinical picture, should also be considered [6, 28].

High inflammatory markers and systemic involvement should also be particularly considered in the differential diagnosis of acute COVID-19 with systemic manifestations. This is because distinguishing MIS-A with multi-organ involvement, which can have both acute and biphasic courses, from both acute COVID-19 and the acute sequelae of SARS-CoV-2 infection can be challenging [14, 17]. While there are some clinical similarities in terms of symptoms and signs between MIS-A and COVID-19, rashes and gastrointestinal symptoms are more commonly seen in MIS-A, whereas upper respiratory symptoms such as cough and runny nose are more pronounced in COVID-19. Since the treatment for these two diseases is different, making the correct differentiation is of vital importance [14].

Due to the severity of the disease and the possibility of rapid progression, the cornerstone of successful treatment for the patient lies in suspecting MIS-A based on the medical history (especially recent recovery from COVID-19) and clinical symptoms, excluding alternative diagnoses, and making an early diagnosis [14].

10. Treatment

MIS-A therapy is generally adapted from the treatment guidelines developed for MIS-C. There is no uniform treatment strategy for MIS-A. Treatment largely focuses on immunosuppression using steroids or other immunomodulators, and supportive therapies (such as fluid resuscitation, inotropic support, and respiratory support) are used in most cases [29]. From a clinical point of view, undetected MIS-A has a high mortality rate [14]. The prognosis of the disease depends on early recognition of the condition and prompt administration of immunomodulatory therapy, which reduces the risk of developing life-threatening complications [6, 30]. The published literature on MIS-A is limited to small case series and a single observational epidemiological study that provides little data to guide treatment decisions for MIS-A patients. Therefore, MIS-A treatment is usually adapted from the treatment guidelines developed for MIS-C [31]. No randomized controlled trials have compared different treatment approaches for MIS-C. However, data from descriptive and observational comparative efficacy studies are available to guide MIS-C treatment [31]. This section summarizes the recommendations of the COVID-19 Treatment Guidelines Panel (NIH, July 21, 2023) for the therapeutic management of pediatric patients with multisystem inflammatory syndrome in children (MIS-C). Includes individuals <21 years of age, according to the Centers for Disease Control and Prevention (CDC) MIS-C case definition [31].

Children with MIS-C are recommended to be treated in centers where a multidisciplinary team consisting of experts in cardiology, hematology, infectious diseases, intensive care, and rheumatology is available when immunomodulatory therapy is applied. Based on previously reported cases, intravenous immunoglobulin (IVIG) and glucocorticoids are the most used immunomodulatory treatments in children with MIS-C. The American College of Rheumatology recommends the combination of IVIG and glucocorticoids as the first-line immunomodulatory treatment for hospitalized children with MIS-C. The NIH (COVID-19 Treatment Guidelines Panel) the panel also suggests the combined use of IVIG and low to moderate-dose glucocorticoids in children hospitalized with MIS-C. The glucocorticoid dose considered low to moderate is typically 1 to 2 mg/kg/day of methylprednisolone or an equivalent dose of another glucocorticoid [31].

The IVIG dose should be administered at a dose of 2 g/kg based on the ideal body weight and should not exceed a maximum total dose of 100 g. During the patient's IVIG infusion, heart function and fluid status should be monitored, and in cases where there is a risk of developing fluid-related issues, the IVIG dose can be divided into 1 g/kg doses based on the ideal body weight and spread over 2 days. When clinical improvement occurs in the patient, glucocorticoid doses should be gradually reduced [31].

In children with MIS-C, the absence of fever, a decrease in inflammatory parameters in laboratory measurements (especially C-reactive protein, CRP, IL-6, sedimentation rate, etc.), and the improvement of end-organ dysfunction are considered as signs of clinical improvement. Studies have shown that the combined use of IVIG and glucocorticoids provides additional benefits compared to monotherapy with glucocorticoids or IVIG alone. Therefore, the NIH recommends IVIG monotherapy as the initial treatment only when steroids are contraindicated, while glucocorticoid monotherapy is recommended in cases where IVIG is not available or contraindicated [31].

10.1 Hospitalized children with treatment-resistant MIS-C may require intensified immunomodulatory therapy

In general, children hospitalized with MIS-C tend to respond well to initial immunomodulatory treatment, with clinical improvement often seen on the first day of treatment. However, some children may not show this clinical improvement and may experience worsening organ dysfunction alongside persistent fever and increased inflammatory markers. In cases where children with MIS-C do not respond to treatment within 24 hours of the initial immunomodulatory therapy, the NIH recommends transitioning to intensified therapy. Response to treatment is considered as the resolution of fever, a decrease in inflammatory markers, and improvement in end-organ dysfunction [31].

For children with NIH-defined treatment-resistant MIS-C, the NIH recommends additional immunomodulatory therapy with anakinra, high-dose glucocorticoids, or infliximab. There is insufficient evidence to determine which of these agents is superior for intensified therapy in treatment-resistant MIS-C. Therefore, they are recommended in alphabetical order [31].

In cases of severe disease resistance, combination therapy with high-dose glucocorticoids and anakinra or high-dose glucocorticoids and infliximab can be used for intensified treatment. However, anakinra and infliximab should not be used in combination. In cases of treatment-resistant MIS-C, intensified therapy with a second dose of IVIG is not recommended by the NIH, especially for cases that did not respond to initial treatment. The NIH emphasizes the high risk of IVIG resistance, concerns about fluid overload, and the potential for rapid disease progression in such cases [31].

Patients receiving immunosuppressive treatment are at a higher risk of infections. The NIH emphasizes that the risks and benefits of using these agents should be evaluated individually for each patient, especially in immunocompromised MIS-C patients, as there is an increased risk of secondary infections with immunomodulatory therapy [31].

In the case of MIS-C, positive results have been observed in patients treated with Intensified Immunomodulatory Therapy using High-Dose Glucocorticoids. High-dose glucocorticoid therapy is defined as the intravenous (IV) administration of 10 to 30 mg/kg/day of methylprednisolone or an equivalent corticosteroid. After 1 to 3 days of high-dose glucocorticoids, the treatment is transitioned to low to moderate doses (1–2 mg/kg/day) [31].

10.2 Anakinra

Anakinra has been used successfully in the treatment of IVIG-resistant Kawasaki disease and is commonly used in other hyperinflammatory syndromes like macrophage activation syndrome in pediatric patients. Anakinra has a good safety record and is the most used biological agent for the treatment of MIS-C in children in the United States. An advantage of anakinra is its short half-life (4–6 hours), allowing it to be quickly discontinued when necessary. High-dose anakinra (5–10 mg/kg/day) is recommended for MIS-C patients based on its proven efficacy in macrophage activation syndrome. The duration of treatment can vary but it has been noted that it can be used as a long-term steroid-sparing agent for up to 2 weeks [31].

NIH recommends Infliximab as an option for intensified treatment in hospitalized MIS-C patients. A single dose of IV Infliximab (5–10 mg/kg) is suggested [31].

Furthermore, there is a consensus among the panel that low-dose aspirin should be given as antithrombotic therapy to MIS-C patients without bleeding risk. It is also noted that antiviral treatment is not expected to be beneficial since MIS-C is thought to develop because of a disrupted immune response weeks after the primary SARS-CoV-2 infection [31].

MIS-C patients are at an increased risk of developing shock, and shock management is recommended to follow the Pediatric Septic Shock Management Guidelines [31].

According to the analysis results by Kunal et al., who investigated the treatment of MIS-A in a total of 79 patients, steroids (60.2%) and intravenous immunoglobulins

DOI: http://dx.doi.org/10.5772/intechopen.1003222

(37.2%) were most often used in the treatment. Only about 10% of patients required biological treatment [18].

According to Patel's study, which included 221 patients, anticoagulant treatment was used in 110 of 193 patients receiving MIS-A treatment, corticosteroids were used in 152 of 205 patients, and IVIG treatment was used in 112 of 205 patients. Immunomodulators were used in 42 of 203 patients. Shock or hypotension developed in 51% of the patients, 115 of the 201 patients were admitted to the intensive care unit, and 15 of the patients (7%) died [15].

11. Conclusion

Multisystem inflammatory syndrome in adults (MIS-A) is a rare and not fully understood post-infection complication of COVID-19, potentially life-threatening, and has been reported in a limited number of cases worldwide. From a clinical perspective, undiagnosed MIS-A has a high mortality rate. The prognosis of the disease relies on early recognition of the condition and the immediate application of immunomodulatory treatments (such as steroids, immunoglobulins, etc.) that reduce the risk of life-threatening complications. Due to the risk of rapidly developing decompensation and critical illness, patients require urgent medical intervention. MIS-A should be considered in cases of sudden cardiac symptoms of unknown cause. Therefore, increasing awareness among clinicians about this emerging disease is essential. More research is needed to better understand the pathophysiology of the multisystem inflammatory syndrome and optimize its treatment.

Author details

Yeter Eylül Bayram
Department of Internal Medicine, Hamidiye Sisli Etfal Training and Research Hospital, Istanbul, Turkey

*Address all correspondence to: ytrbayram@hotmail.com

References

[1] Lin YF, Duan Q, Zhou Y, et al. Spread and impact of COVID-19 in China: A systematic review and synthesis of predictions from transmission-dynamic models. Frontiers in Medicine (Lausanne). 2020;**7**:321

[2] Mieczkowska K, Zhu TH, Hoffman L, et al. Two adult cases of multisystem inflammatory syndrome associated with SARS-CoV-2. JAAD Case Reports. 2021;**10**:113-115

[3] Ni W, Yang X, Yang D, et al. Role of angiotensin-converting enzyme 2 (ACE2) in COVID-19. Critical Care. 2020;**24**:422

[4] Aziz M, Brenner M, Wang P. Therapeutic potential of B-1a cells in COVID-19. Shock. 2020;**54**:586-594

[5] Baj J, Karakuła-Juchnowicz H, Teresiński G, et al. COVID-19: Specific and non-specific clinical manifestations and symptoms: The current state of knowledge. Journal of Clinical Medicine. 2020;**9**:1753

[6] Bayram YE, Yildiz-Sevgi D, Yavuz A, Cancetin M, Gurler MY. Management skin manifestation of multisystem inflammatory syndrome associated with SARS-CoV-2. Virology Journal. 2022;**19**:9

[7] Mahajan P, Dass B, Radhakrishnan N, McCullough PA. COVID-19-associated systemic thromboembolism: A case report and review of the literature. Cardiorenal Medicine. 2020;**10**:462-469

[8] Hoste L, Van Paemel R, Haerynck F. Multisystem inflammatory syndrome in children related to COVID-19: A systematic review. European Journal of Pediatrics. 2021;**180**:2019-2034

[9] Graciano-Machuca O, Villegas-Rivera G, López-Pérez I, Macías-Barragán J, Sifuentes-Franco S. Multisystem inflammatory syndrome in children (MIS-C) following SARS-CoV-2 infection: Role of oxidative stress. Frontiers in Immunology. 2021;**12**:723654

[10] Rafferty MS, Burrows H, Joseph JP, Leveille J, Nihtianova S, Amirian ES. Multisystem inflammatory syndrome in children (MIS-C) and the coronavirus pandemic: Current knowledge and implications for public health. Journal of Infection and Public Health. 2021;**14**:484-494

[11] Tam H, El Tal T, Go E, Yeung RSM. Pediatric inflammatory multisystem syndrome temporally associated with COVID-19: A spectrum of diseases with many names. CMAJ. 2020;**192**:E1093-E10e6

[12] Ahmad F, Ahmed A, Rajendraprasad SS, et al. Multisystem inflammatory syndrome in adults: A rare sequela of SARS-CoV-2 infection. International Journal of Infectious Diseases. 2021;**108**:209-211

[13] Huynh T, Sanchez-Flores X, Yau J, Huang JT. Cutaneous manifestations of SARS-CoV-2 infection. American Journal of Clinical Dermatology. 2022;**23**:277-286

[14] Zahornacky O, Porubčin Š, Rovnakova A, Jarcuska P. Multisystem inflammatory syndrome in adults associated with recent infection with COVID-19. Diagnostics (Basel). 2023;**13**(5):983

[15] Patel P, DeCuir J, Abrams J, Campbell AP, Godfred-Cato S, Belay ED. Clinical characteristics of multisystem inflammatory syndrome in adults:

A systematic review. JAMA Network Open. 2021;**4**:e2126456

[16] Melgar M, Haston J, DeCuir J, et al. Multisystem inflammatory syndrome in adults: Case finding through systematic review of electronic medical records. Clinical Infectious Diseases. 2022;**75**:1903-1911

[17] Morris SB, Schwartz NG, Patel P, et al. Case series of multisystem inflammatory syndrome in adults associated with SARS-CoV-2 infection —United Kingdom and United States, March-August 2020. MMWR. Morbidity and Mortality Weekly Report. 2020;**69**:1450-1456

[18] Kunal S, Ish P, Sakthivel P, Malhotra N, Gupta K. The emerging threat of multisystem inflammatory syndrome in adults (MIS-A) in COVID-19: A systematic review. Heart & Lung. 2022;**54**:7-18

[19] Caterson HC, Xu G, Adelstein S, Puranik R. A diagnosis that a cardiologist should not MIS: Multisystem inflammatory syndrome in adults. Heart, Lung & Circulation. 2022;**31**:1706-1709

[20] Gawas A, Nevrekar RP, Khandeparkar AV. Multiorgan inflammatory syndrome in adults MIS-A post SARS-CoV-2 infection: A novel clinical enigma. The Journal of the Association of Physicians of India. 2023;**71**:11-12

[21] Yao Q, Waley L, Liou N. Adult presentation of multisystem inflammatory syndrome (MIS) associated with recent COVID-19 infection: Lessons learnt in timely diagnosis and management. BML Case Reports. 2021;**14**:e243114

[22] Belay ED, Godfred Cato S, Rao AK, et al. Multisystem inflammatory syndrome in adults after severe acute respiratory syndrome coronavirus 2 (SARS-CoV-2) infection and coronavirus disease 2019 (COVID-19) vaccination. Clinical Infectious Diseases. 2022;**75**:e741-e7e8

[23] Vogel TP, Top KA, Karatzios C, et al. Multisystem inflammatory syndrome in children and adults (MIS-C/A): Case definition & guidelines for data collection, analysis, and presentation of immunization safety data. Vaccine. 2021;**39**:3037-3049

[24] Multisystem Inflammatory Syndrome in Adults (MIS-A) Case Definition and Information for Healthcare Providers. Available from: https://www.cdc.gov/mis/mis-a/hcp.html#:~:text=CDC%20Case%20Definition%20for%20MIS%2DA&text=Subjective%20fever%20or%20documented%20fever,first%20THREE%20days%20of%20hospitalization*

[25] Chuang YY, Huang YC, Lin TY. Toxic shock syndrome in children: Epidemiology, pathogenesis, and management. Paediatric Drugs. 2005;7:11-25

[26] Holstein B. Multisystem inflammatory syndrome in children. The Journal for Nurse Practitioners. 2021;**17**:941-945

[27] Rajasekaran K, Duraiyarasan S, Adefuye M, Manjunatha N, Ganduri V. Kawasaki disease and coronary artery involvement: A narrative review. Cureus. 2022;**14**:e28358

[28] Shiohara T, Mizukawa Y. Drug-induced hypersensitivity syndrome (DiHS)/drug reaction with eosinophilia and systemic symptoms (DRESS): An update in 2019. Allergology International. 2019;**68**:301-308

[29] Mahmoud S, El-Kalliny M, Kotby A, El-Ganzoury M, Fouda E, Ibrahim H. Treatment of MIS-C in children and adolescents. Current Pediatrics Reports. 2022;**10**:1-10

[30] Duarte R, Cisneros S, Fernandez G, Castellon D, Cattani C, Melo CA, et al. Kawasaki disease: A review with emphasis on cardiovascular complications. Insights Into Imaging. 2010;**1**:223-231

[31] Therapeutic Management of Hospitalized Children With MIS-C, Plus a Discussion on MIS-A. 2023. Available from: https://www.covid19treatmentguidelines.nih.gov/management/clinical-management-of-children/hospitalized-children-therapeutic-management-of-mis-c/

Chapter 2

Omicron: A SARS-CoV-2 Variant

Khushi Gandhi

Abstract

COVID-19 is a viral disease caused by SARS-CoV-2. Various variants of SARS-CoV-2 were responsible for causing havoc worldwide resulting in approximately 6.9 million deaths across the globe to date. Since the end of 2021, Omicron (B.1.1.529) has been the recent most variant to be studied and understood to a greater extent. Omicron was found to be the most mutated variant, which enhanced its pathogenic characteristics. Its highly contagious nature and the ability to evade immunity have made it a cause of global concern. The variant also poses a serious risk of reinfection. Furthermore, vaccines developed in response to COVID-19 were found to be less successful with Omicron infections. For the development of targeted vaccines and efficient therapeutic methods, it is necessary to understand the pathogenesis of Omicron. Numerous studies have been conducted to analyze the molecular properties of this variant. This chapter summarizes the biological and molecular properties of this variant and its successive mutations. Further, the clinical traits of the variant, including its pathogenicity, transmissibility and response to body's immune actions and vaccines are discussed. Precisely examining the mechanisms through which the variant infects and propagates inside the host can aid in preventing the illness and lead to successful management of its global spread.

Keywords: Omicron, SARS-CoV-2, COVID-19, mutation, transmission, pathogenicity, immune evasion

1. Introduction

Coronavirus disease (COVID-19) caused by the severe acute respiratory syndrome coronavirus 2 (SARS-CoV-2) first emerged in Wuhan, China in December 2019. The patients infected with virus showed symptoms similar to severe acute respiratory syndrome (SARS) and Middle East respiratory syndrome (MERS), including cough, fever and chest discomfort. In January 2020, the whole genome sequence was performed on the novel coronavirus. The outbreak then reached its peak in China in February and later spread worldwide [1, 2]. Since then, there have been 770+ million confirmed cases and 6.9 million deaths globally [3]. Coronaviruses are RNA viruses belonging to the family *Coronaviridae* and order *Nidovirales*. *Nidovirales* are known to have large genomes, high replicative rate and exhibit various enzymatic activities [2].

Mutations are a natural phenomenon commonly seen during the course of replication. SARS-CoV-2 has a great capacity of undergoing mutations and resulting in antigenic changes over time. It is known to evolve at the rate of one substitution approximately every 11 days [4]. New variants of SARS-CoV-2 have hence emerged through accumulation of these mutations. These variations, however, contribute to increased transmissibility, disease progression and reduced treatment efficacy among other concerns [5]. Specific strains of SARS-CoV-2 have been declared as variants of concern (VOC) due to their highly infectious nature and ability to cause re-infections. These VOCs tend to have mutations that lead to alterations in receptor binding, higher transmissibility, reduced antibody neutralization, decreased therapeutic effects and potentially increased disease severity [6].

The first emerged VOC of SARS-CoV-2 is the Alpha (B.1.1.7) variant. It was first detected in the UK in September 2020. It showcased 14 non-synonymous mutations and three deletions. Eight of these were on the spike protein, resulting in increased affinity towards the ACE2 receptors through which the virus entered the host's cells. The variant also showed higher viral load and mortality [4, 5, 7]. The Beta (B.1.351) variant was the next VOC, emerging in South Africa in October 2020. It too possessed nine mutations on the spike protein, with three being on the receptor binding domain (RBD). It exhibited increased transmissibility; however, similar effects were not seen in terms of disease severity and fatality [7–9]. The Gamma (P.1 or B.1.1.28), first detected in Brazil in January 2021, showed 10 mutations on the spike protein, with three on the RBD. The gamma variant significantly reduced treatment efficiency with previously used monoclonal antibody (mAb) cocktail showing reduced neutralization [5, 8, 10]. Fourth VOC of SARS-CoV-2—the Delta (B.1.617.2) emerged in India in May 2021. It had several mutations at the spike protein. Interestingly, along with the RBD, N-terminal domain (NTD) region of the spike protein also showed numerous amino acid alterations. This was not seen in the earlier variants. The Delta variant too showed reduced susceptibility to priorly used antibodies and exhibited a high transmissibility rate [8, 11, 12].

Omicron (B.1.1.529) is the recent most VOC of SARS-CoV-2. It was first reported in South Africa in November 2021. Omicron exhibited far more mutations than any other variant that emerged before it. It also demonstrated a very high transmission rate and by the beginning of December, it had spread worldwide, becoming the dominant variant of SARS-CoV-2. It contributed to 99.7% of the confirmed cases in the months of February and March 2022. Omicron could not only successfully escape immunological responses but also alter them. Antibodies formed from previous infections or vaccines offered little to no protection against the variant. Moreover, Omicron posed a high risk of reinfection. The only relief was the reduced severity of

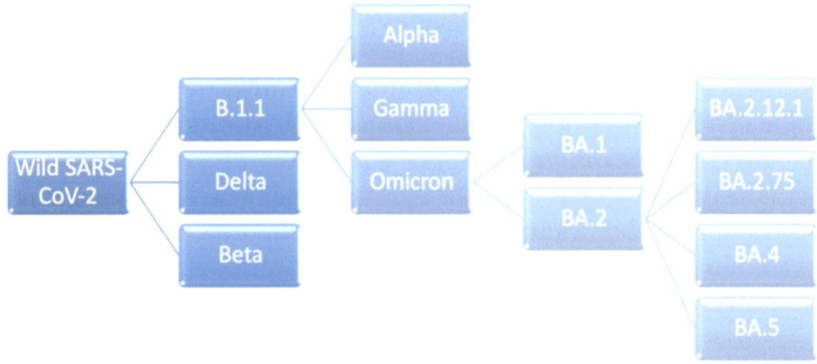

Figure 1.
Evolution of the VoCs of SARS-CoV-2. Mutations in the structural proteins, especially S protein of the SARS-CoV-2 led to the emergence of different variants, which because of their threatening nature, were titled variants of concern. SARS-CoV-2, severe acute respiratory syndrome [17].

illness and hence reduced mortality. Over time, sub-variants of Omicron too emerged [4, 13–16]. Specific mutations on structural proteins enabled Omicron to exhibit such attributes. Omicron's molecular structure, mutations and pathogenic traits are discussed in detail later (**Figure 1**).

2. Omicron at the molecular level

The novel Beta coronavirus, SARS-CoV-2, is an enveloped virus with a single-stranded RNA as the genetic material [18, 19]. It primarily consists of four structural proteins—the membrane (M) protein, the envelope (E) protein, the spike (S) protein and the nucleocapsid (N) protein [20, 21]. The E protein aids in the formation of pentameric ion channels in the virus's body while the M protein acts as the fundamental structural protein [20, 22]. The N protein plays an essential role in the packaging of the viral RNA in the helical nucleocapsid and formation of the liquid enveloped. It further interacts with the other structural proteins during virion assembly and aids in the virus's replication [21]. S protein is made up of two subunits—S1 (head) and S2 (stem) [20, 22].

It is the S protein that plays the central role in the binding of the virus with the host's ACE2 receptors, causing the integration of the membranes of the virus and the host cell [20]. The M protein, through the association with the host's endoplasmic reticulum, aids in the formation of viral particles, which is performed by the virus's RNA by using the host's resources [23]. Thus, the structural proteins (found in the spike, membrane, envelope and the nucleocapsid) contribute to the virulence of SARS-CoV-2 and aid in higher pathogenicity and infectivity [5]. Other than this, the viral genome codes for 16 non-structural and 9 accessory proteins. The non-structural proteins (NSPs) are involved in the replication and translation of the viral RNA while the accessory proteins (ORFs 3a, 3b, 6, 7a, 7b, 8, 9b, 9c and 10) regulate the virus's interaction with the host and aid in immunity evasion and virulence enhancement [20, 24].

The Omicron variant (B.1.1.529) of SARS-CoV-2, upon genome sequence analysis, was found to have numerous synonymous and non-synonymous mutations [25]. It has been the most mutated variant reported to date, with more than 60 substitutions, deletions and insertions [5, 26]. Most of the mutations were observed in the S protein—with 28 amino acid substitutions, 3 deletions and 1 insertion in the Omicron 21 K lineage [16, 26, 27]. The key mutations in the spike protein are: A67V, del69–70, T95I, del142–144, Y145D, del211, L212I, ins214 EPE, G339D, S371L, S373P, S375F, K417N, N440K, G446S, S477N, T478K, E484A, Q493R, G496S, Q498R, N501Y, Y505H, T547K, D614G, H655Y, N679K, P681H, N764K, D796Y, N856K, Q954H, N969K, L981F [16, 25]. **Figure 2** illustrates the mutations observed in the proteins of the Omicron variant.

These mutations in the S protein have been correlated with disease severity, infectivity and immune evasion [5]. Two mutations have been associated with S protein's enhanced affinity to ACE2 receptors, thus improving the virus's attachment to the host cell. Three mutations near the cleavage site may aid in boosting Omicron's transmissibility [16, 28]. Moreover, 15 of these mutations have been discovered to be in the RBD (residues 319–541), which is the key target of the neutralizing antibodies (nAb) [16, 25, 29]. However, some studies showed that the current nAb will still bind with the mutated spike protein and the mutated RBD of Omicron had a low predisposition towards the antibodies. Hence, antibodies produced by previous SARS-CoV-2 infections or vaccines may still offer some protection against the Omicron variant [16, 30]. Interestingly Omicron

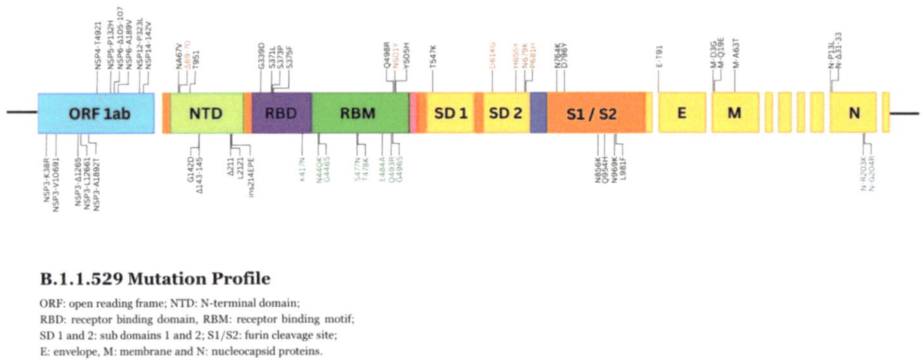

Figure 2.
Omicron (B.1.1.529) mutation profile. S protein was found to be heavily mutated. Mutations depicted in red are known to enhance the binding affinity with ACE2 receptors, resulting in an increase in the infectivity of the variant. Mutations in green aid in immune evasion while mutations in blue promote viral replication leading to a high viral load and virulence. ORF, open reading frame; NTD, N-terminal domain; RBD, receptor binding domain; RBM, receptor binding motif; SD 1 and 2, sub-domains 1 and 2; S1/S2, Furin cleavage site; E, envelope; M, membrane; N, Nucleocapsid proteins [25].

exhibited no mutations in the accessory proteins, which are immunological regulators and are often heavily altered. This indicated the selection pressures on Omicron [31]. Further, while comparing the nucleotide changes in Omicron with other variants, Alpha variant was found to be the closest with an identity percentage of 99.63% [16, 32].

2.1 Subvariants of Omicron

Omicron is further classified into four sub-strains by WHO—BA.1, BA.1.1, BA.2 and BA.3. Each sub-strain has different properties with respect to their transmissibility, pathogenicity, growth and infectivity. BA.1 and BA.2 have significant differences in their mutations contributing to virulent attributes. Out of the two, BA.2 is the more transmittable (33% higher rate) and has a significant growth advantage. Five different mutations in the RBD of the spike protein are responsible for this

Attributes		**BA.1 Sub-variant**	**BA.2 Sub-variant**
Unique mutations in the S protein	RBD region	G496S	T376A, D405N, R408S,
	Non-RBD region	A67V, HV69-, T95I, VYY143-, NL211I, 215EPE, T547K, N856K, L981F	T19I, LPP24-26-/ A27S, V213G,
Transmissibility and infectivity		Lower	Higher (33%)
Replication efficacy		Lower	Higher (1.4-fold)
Pathogenicity		Lower	Higher
Case severity		Similar	
Therapeutic and vaccine efficacy		Similar	

Certain differences in the mutations on the S protein of the sub-variants were observed, which resulted in differences in specific characteristics. This included a higher infectivity rate and pathogenicity in BA.2 sub-variant. However, both the sub-variants resulted in similar severity in cases and had a similar response against various vaccines and treatments [35–38].

Table 1.
Comparative analysis between the Omicron sub-variants BA.1 and BA.2.

enhancement [5, 33, 34]. **Table 1** summarizes and compares the key characteristics of BA.1 and BA.2 sub-variants.

Even though all the sub-variants emerged around the same time, BA.1 dominated the cases worldwide. The reason still remains unclear, although some researchers attribute this to the spike protein variations, which regulate the virus's entry into the host cell and its further propagation [39]. BA.3 has been predominantly observed in hospitalized patients, indicating higher disease severity. However, it caused the lowest number of cases out of the three [40]. BA.4 and BA.5 have also been identified as Omicron sub-variants [41]. All these variants are under study to understand the immunological resilience of Omicron [5].

3. Transmission of Omicron

SARS-CoV-2 transmits primarily through two methods—direct viral spread or droplet infection [5]. Omicron, similar to the other variants, infects the host cells in the similar fashion. However, it has a greater infectivity rate [27]. Numerous studies reported its high transmissibility, for instance, a study from South Africa reported doubling times of 3.38 d, while a study from the UK reported doubling times of 2–2.5 d, with the basic reproduction number more than 3 [42–44]. With respect to the Delta variant, Omicron is reported to have a 3.2 times higher transmission rate, with an average of 3 days as the doubling time [35, 45]. The mutations in the spike protein have been thought to contribute in making Omicron extremely contagious [16].

Various pieces of evidence have been provided by different studies to substantiate the above-made claim. For instance, an *in vitro* Chinese study used an AI model to show that the mutations at locations N440K, N501Y and T478K directly contributed to increased infectivity, with tenfold increase in Omicron with respect to the original SARS-CoV-2 variation and a double increase with respect to the Delta variant [46]. Another study found the combination of mutations N501Y and Q498R significantly enhance the S protein's binding affinity to the ACE2 receptors [47]. Other mutations such as the N679K, D614G and P681H have also been associated with higher infectivity [16, 48].

4. Pathogenicity of Omicron

SARS-CoV-2 infects humans through different cell types of the respiratory system such as the airway and alveolar epithelium cells, the vascular endothelial cells, etc. by binding to the ACE2 receptor [5, 49]. This binding, as discussed earlier, is facilitated by the spike protein. Studies even found high Omicron infection in cells possessing high number of ACE2 receptors [50]. However, Omicron has been found to follow a different route. Omicron enters through the endosomal pathway, instead of the plasma membrane followed by the other variants. This pathway is enhanced by cathepsins instead of TMPRSS2 [51, 52].

A study found that the infection by Omicron was more significant in the cells, which exhibited a lower TMPRSS2 expression. This further indicated that Omicron followed the endosomal entry pathway [53]. This altered entry pathway has been associated with better success in the virus's replication in the upper respiratory tract [54]. Omicron has also been observed to have a lower cleavage efficiency in comparison to the other emerged variants such as the Gamma and the Alpha variant. Mutations like the N679K and H655Y are the primary cause of the same [35, 55].

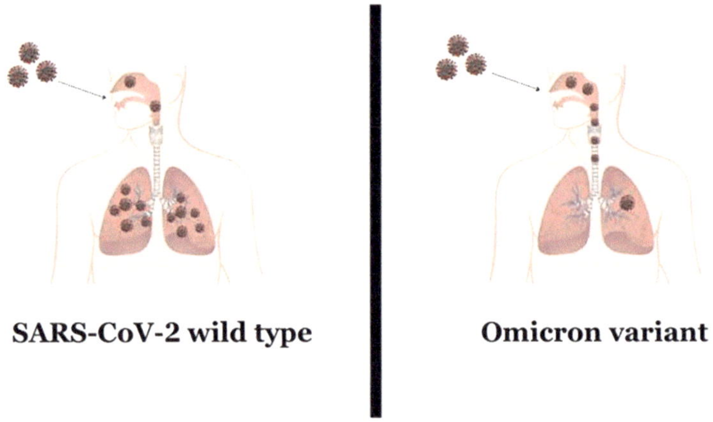

Figure 3.
Comparison of observed viral load in omicron with the SARS-CoV-2 wild type. The Omicron variant tends to accumulate in the upper respiratory tract, exhibiting higher viral load in the nasal region and larynx. While, the SARS-Cov-2 wild type as well as the other variants settle in the lower respiratory tract, resulting in a higher viral load in the lungs. SARS-CoV-2, severe acute respiratory syndrome [35].

Other mutations in the N and S proteins have been linked to the variant's enhanced cellular permeability. These mutations also aid in more efficient capsid assembly, found to be three-fold better than the Delta variant [56]. The sub-variants of Omicron (BA.1 and BA.2) do not form syncytia (normally produced at the boundary of S1 and S2 during the processing of the S protein), owing to the numerous changes in the S protein. These alterations, combined with the altered entry pathway result in different cellular tropism [35, 54].

Viral load may also be associated with Omicron's high transmissibility and growth rate. A higher viral load was reported in the upper airway (specifically the nose, trachea and throat). This aggregation of the viral particles in the upper respiratory tract may result from higher growth and increased viral load [35]. **Figure 3** illustrates the difference in observed viral load in Omicron in comparison to the other variants.

Omicron also has the ability to cause reinfection [42]. Data from South Africa showed that the reinfection rates increased significantly during the Omicron wave in comparison to the Beta and Delta waves [57]. In the UK, it was reported that there was 6 times higher risk of reinfection with Omicron with respect to the Delta variant. A prior COVID-19 infection provided 80% protection against the Delta variant, however, only 19% protection was observed against the Omicron variant [44]. The good news is that fewer cases of Omicron infections required hospitalization, while the frequency of severe cases was more in Alpha and Delta infections [25].

5. Body's response to infection

Upon infection with SARS-CoV-2, the innate immune cells, primarily consisting of the neutrophils and the macrophages, identify the virus and activate the immune response. Cytokines and chemokines such as Interleukin-6 (IL-6), monocyte chemoattractant protein-1 and Interferon γ (IFN-γ) are then secreted by these immune cells. Monocytes, neutrophils and macrophages, attracted by the released chemicals, reach the site of infection and release cytotoxic chemicals to kill the virus. The virus is fought by cytotoxic CDB+ T cells, CD4+ T helper cells and B cells. The CDB+ T cells eradicate the virus through cytotoxins while the B cells produce nAb. The cellular reaction is efficient and long-lasting and also triggers immuno-protective memory [5, 58–61]. A study identified the 14 neutralizing IgG antibodies from SARS-CoV-2 infected patients, with BD-368-2 being the most potent [62]. Other antibodies recovered were IgI and IgM. These antibodies were specific to RBD suggesting that anti-RBD antibodies can be used as clinical interventions against SARS-CoV-2 infections [63].

The Omicron variant triggers exactly the same immune reactions as that seen in the wild type of SARS-CoV-2 variant. The infection results in the production of cytotoxic and follicular T helper cells, along with RBD and spike-related IgG+ B cells and memory B cells. The cytotoxic T cells - CDB+ T cells produce proteases and induce apoptosis in infected cells. On the other hand, the B cells derived from the pool of live memory cells interact with the spike protein [5, 35, 53, 64].

5.1 Clinical manifestations of Omicron

Clinical symptoms of the Omicron infection were different from the earlier variants. Most prevalent symptoms included a cough, nasal congestion, sore throat and fatigue. Loss of smell and taste, fever, dizziness, headaches, etc. were less prevalent with respect to the Delta variant [65, 66]. The virus also affects the organs, which extensively express ACE2 such as glandular cells of the gastric, duodenal and rectal epithelium [67]. A study found that the acute symptoms lasted for fewer days in the Omicron outbreak with an average of 6.87 days, while during the Delta wave, they lasted for an average of 8.89 days [68]. Omicron infection was also suggested to exhibit milder symptoms with a lot of the cases being asymptomatic and majority requiring no hospitalization. In total, 2.6% of the Delta variant infected patients were admitted to hospitals while only 1.9% of Omicron-infected patients required hospitalization [35, 68, 69]. A study found that out of the Omicron-infected individuals, 36.1% did not exhibit any antibody response, while 62.7% produced IgG and only 1.2% produced IgM along with IgG [70]. Omicron-infected patients exhibited various hematological disorders such as lymphocytopenia, neutrophilia, anemia, erythrocytopenia, thrombocytopenia etc. These can be used as biomarkers in Omicron infections for a better prognosis [71].

5.2 Severe cases of Omicron infection

In vivo investigations revealed that lower viral load, smaller lung damage and lower mortality rates were observed in Omicron infections in comparison to the other variants [72, 73]. As discussed earlier, the viral load tends to settle in the upper respiratory tract and not so much in the lungs [74]. However, severe cases of Omicron can result in pneumonia and respiratory failure and can even be fatal [75, 76]. Significant comorbidities, including hypertension, bronchitis and diabetes, have been observed in Omicron infections [35].

The major damage to the tissues in COVID-19, however, is caused majorly by the host's immune reactions and not directly by the virus itself. The host's immune reactions are crucial in the pathophysiology of COVID-19 and are directly connected with the disease's progression. Severe SARS-CoV-2 infections have been shown to dysregulate the host's normal immune responses. As discussed earlier, the infection leads to numerous hematological disorders such as leukocytosis, lymphocytopenia and a high neutrophil-lymphocyte ratio (NLR). This is the first sign of immunological dysregulation, resulting in uncontrolled inflammatory reactions. These processes lead to immune cells' damage and exaggerated responses by macrophages, eventually resulting in cell death and tissue damage due to the release of cytotoxic substances. Its manifestations are also seen as cytokine storms and organ failures [5, 71, 77–79].

Cytokine release syndrome (CRS) is often observed in severe cases of COVID-19. CRS is a hyperinflammatory condition resulting from augmented release of inflammatory cytokines such as tumor necrosis factor (TNF), IL -1, –6, –12, –18, – 33 and IFN -I and -II, along with certain chemokines, including CCL -2, –3, –5 and CXCL -8, –9, 10 [77, 80, 81]. CRS results in acute respiratory distress syndrome, characterized by alveolar epithelial and endothelial destruction in lungs followed by breathing difficulty, hypoxemia and pulmonary oedema. This causes organ failure and also becomes fatal in severe cases [5, 82, 83].

5.3 Immune evasion by Omicron

Omicron has exhibited the ability to alter the host's immune responses. Some mutations enable the variant to weaken the T cells' capacity to identify and destroy the infected cells. In some instances, Omicron has also been observed to escape the nAb produced from previous infections or vaccines. However, the existing nAb still provides protection against severe illnesses [16, 84, 85]. Certain viral proteins such as the Orf3 and Orf6 were also observed to alter the T cell responses, which affected the IFN activations. Omicron also brought on T cell immunity decline through immunological fatigue and memory deficits. All this resulted in easier reproduction and propagation of the variant [16, 86, 87].

The understanding of the immunopathogenesis of SARS-CoV-2 aided in developing efficient treatment therapies. However, the precise mechanisms through which the Omicron infection progresses are unclear. For the development of Omicron-specific immunological therapies, it is necessary to analyze the distinct pathophysiology during Omicron infections [5, 88].

6. Omicron diagnosis

Provisionally, the infection can be diagnosed according to the symptoms. It is confirmed using reverse transcription polymerase chain reaction (RT-PCR) or other nucleic acid tests. Serological assays can be used to detect a past infection. They detect the antibodies that were produced by the body in response to the infection. Other laboratory tests can further help in detecting the severity of the infection such as lactate dehydrogenase (LDH), C-reactive protein (CRP), ferritin and IL-6 levels. Along with laboratory testing, chest CT scans may be helpful to diagnose COVID-19 in individuals with a high clinical suspicion of infection [89, 90].

For the Omicron variant, RT-PCR still remains the gold standard. The RT-PCR diagnostics kits primarily focus on the E, Rp, Rd. and N genes. The S gene mutation observed in the case of Omicron variant may or may not cause a positive test [5, 91, 92]. To identify and classify the variant, next generation sequencing (NGS) is required. NGS also aids in determining the origin of SARS-CoV-2. It also has the opportunity to rebuild whole viral genomes. However, unlike PCR, NGS is expensive, time-consuming and requires expertise for interpretation [5, 93, 94]. Serological assays use S or N protein-specific antibodies. These assays also provide insights into the disease severity—with higher amounts of IgG, IgM and IgI antibodies being reported in severe cases [95].

7. Omicron treatment and prevention

Important therapeutics for SARS-CoV-2 infection were mAb cocktails such as casirivimab-imdevimab, bamlanivimab-etesevimab that aided in preventing severe disease or hospitalization. These antibodies target the spike protein for neutralization because, as stated before, it is the spike protein that is responsible for the virus's entry into the host cells by binding to the ACE2 receptors. However, 15 key mutations in the RBD area on the S protein in the Omicron variant may prevent the antibodies from binding with the virus [16, 42]. RBS-A, RBS-B, RBS-C, CR302 and S309 are some of the key targets of the nAb which were replaced in the Omicron variant [96]. This caused scientists worldwide to question the efficacy of such antibodies. *In vitro* studies too suggested that the Omicron variant is successful in completely escaping neutralization by these antibodies. Nevertheless, mAbs that target sites beyond the RBD, such as sotrovimab and cilgavimab/tixagevimab, have been reported to still remain effective against Omicron in similar studies. Another authorized mAb—bebtelovimab too retained its *in vitro* activity against the Omicron sub-strains BA.1 and BA.2 [16, 42, 97–99].

Other antiviral options have also been inspected for emergency use in severe Omicron cases to reduce mortality. Some antivirals proposed are Molnupiravir, Remdesivir, Ensovibep and Camostat. Upon assessment of the above-mentioned and other antiviral molecules against Omicron and its sub-variants, three compounds were found to be particularly efficient. They were Remdesivir, Lufotrelvir and Molnupiravir. Currently, the best antiviral option against omicron is a combination of Nirmatrelvir-Ritonavir. Numerous studies have corroborated the same by analyzing its activity against the variant [35, 100].

7.1 Booster vaccines

The proposal of using booster vaccines was first suggested when *in vitro* studies found an increase of neutralizing antibody titers against omicron in the serum of individuals provided with the booster dose. Vaccines like BNT162B2/mRNA-1273 (Moderna) and Ad26.COV2.S vaccines were given as boosters which resulted in increase of the nAb titers from 122-fold/44-fold lower against omicron to 4–/sixfold lower. Simultaneously, half of the population in the UK were also given booster doses. These booster doses aided in increasing the vaccine's effectiveness against symptomatic infections. They also helped in bringing down severe cases, which required hospitalization. Usually, the nAb response used to wane after a couple of months after the second does. This was restored by the booster vaccine [35, 101, 102].

The Technical Advisory Group on COVID-19 Vaccine Composition (TAG-CO-VAC) advised on globalized access of existing COVID-19 vaccines for booster doses, in light of the transmission of Omicron Variant of Concern (VOC). They suggested the vaccine makers to generate and share data on the vaccine's efficacy against the Omicron variant specifically, along with the other variants. To make the booster doses effective and timely available, the TAG-CO-VAC authorities collaborated with WHO and its expert groups [16].

7.2 Need for new vaccines

As discussed earlier, the Omicron variant is known to escape the mAb, which was effective against the previous variants. Individuals without the booster dose were not able to protect themselves against the variant. Moreover, the booster vaccine also only provided partial protection against it. This indicated the decreasing efficacy of the existing vaccines. Prevalent mutations in Omicron such as Q498R, S477N, Y505H, G496H, T478K, N501Y and E484K are primarily responsible for altering the antigenicity and providing the variant with the capability to evade immune responses. The extensive alterations on the S protein induce stearic hindrance, which in turn affect the antigen–antibody binding. Further, these alterations are unprecedented, making antigen recognition difficult for the antibodies [35, 103–105].

Hence, several researchers advocated the need for development of novel vaccines, particularly targeting the Omicron variant. Numerous vaccines, predominantly bivalent and RNA vaccines, have since been developed by different researchers or pharmacological companies [17, 35]. A few of the clinical trials working on Omicron vaccines are summarized in **Table 2**.

These vaccines show potential in providing protection against Omicron and its sub-variants. Currently, they are under clinical trials for safety and efficacy testing. Numerous studies are under different phases of trials to create a potent vaccine which not only offers protection against the omicron variant but also prevents the need for booster doses [16, 35].

S.No.	Biological interventions	Country of origin	Phase	Clinical trial number	Study title
1	Comirnaty® BNT162b2/Omicron BA.4-5 vaccine (Pfizer-BioNTech) VidPrevtyn® Beta vaccine (Sanofi/GSK)	France	III	NCT05749926	Immunogenicity and Reactogenicity of the Beta-variant Recombinant Protein Booster Vaccine (VidPrevtyn Beta, Sanofi) Compared to a Bivalent mRNA Vaccine (Comirnaty Original/Omicron BA.4-5, BioNTech-Pfizer) in Adults Previously Vaccinated With at Least 3 Doses of COVID-19 mRNA Vaccine
2	Omicron COVID-19 Vaccine (Vero Cell), Inactivated COVID-19 Vaccine (Vero Cell), Inactivated	China	III	NCT05374954	Study on Sequential Immunization of Omicron Inactivated COVID-19 Vaccine and Prototype Inactivated COVID-19 Vaccine in Population Aged 18 Years Old and Above
3	Bivalent BNT162b2 mRNA original/omicron BA.4-5 vaccine Quadrivalent influenza vaccine	Republic of Korea	IIII	NCT05970887	Immunogenicity and Safety of Concomitant Administration of Bivalent COVID-19 Vaccines With Influenza Vaccines
4	Drug: NVX-CoV2515 Drug: NVX-Cov2373 Drug: NVX-CoV2373+NVX-CoV2515 Drug: NVX-CoV2540 Drug: NVX-CoV2373+NVX-CoV2540	Australia	III	NCT05372588	Phase 3 Boosting Study for the SARS-CoV-2 rS Variant Vaccines

S.No.	Biological interventions	Country of origin	Phase	Clinical trial number	Study title
5	BIBP Omicron Inactivated COVID-19 vaccine WIBP Omicron Inactivated COVID-19 vaccine (Vero Cell) COVID-19 Vaccine (Vero Cell), Inactivated	Hong Kong	III	NCT05382871	Sequential Immunization of Two Doses of Inactivated COVID-19 Vaccine (Omicron) in Vaccinated Population Aged 18 Years and Above
6	SCTV01C SCTV01E Sinopharm inactivated COVID-19 vaccine Comirnaty	UAE	III	NCT05323461	A Study to Evaluate the Immunogenicity and Safety of Two Recombinant Protein COVID-19 Vaccines in Population Aged ≥18 Years as Booster Vaccines
7	ABO1020 Placebo	Indonesia	II / III	NCT05636319	A Study to Evaluate the Efficacy, Safety, and Immunogenicity of SARS-CoV-2 Variant (BA.4 /5) mRNA Vaccine
8	BNT162b2 vaccine	Israel	IV	NCT05231005	Fourth BNT162b2 COVID-19 Vaccine Dose
9	mRNA1273 vaccine	Israel	III	NCT05230953	Fourth COVID-19 Vaccine Dose- mRNA1273
10	mRNA-1273 Placebo mRNA-1273.222	USA	II /III	NCT04649151	A Study to Evaluate the Safety, Reactogenicity, and Effectiveness of mRNA-1273 Vaccine in Adolescents 12 to <18 Years Old to Prevent COVID-19

Table 2.
Phase III and IV clinical trials studying novel vaccines against the omicron variant. All of these studies are currently active and not recruiting [106].

8. Conclusion and future prospects

The COVID-19 pandemic resulted in a global public health emergency. The virus's capability to mutate and evolve rapidly became a threatening concern. To keep up with the pace of the virus, the scientific community had to work round the clock for better diagnosis, precise vaccines and treatment methods. While the new Omicron variant exhibited a reduced disease severity, it posed its own set of challenges. Higher transmissibility, increased infectious rate, immune evasion and partial resistance to monoclonal as well as vaccine-induced antibodies are the key challenges that were to be faced. These complications necessitated the development of new technology and alternate approaches to eradicate the virus.

New variants of SARS-CoV-2 were expected to emerge and the virus is still mutating, each time presenting new risks and challenges. Only traditional approaches are not enough to face this challenge, alternate methods have to be incorporated such as the use of bioinformatics and nanotechnology for development of better drugs and/or vaccines. New data are being generated every day by numerous ongoing studies;

however, data interpretation and application require time. Persistent and continued research is necessary for a better understanding of the pathogenesis of the new variants, which will eventually lead to the development of efficient preventive and treatment methods.

Acknowledgements

I would like to acknowledge my professors and mentors, especially Dr. Gayatri Sharma at Amity Institute of Biotechnology, Amity University, Noida, India for their guidance and counsel that helped in completing this chapter.

Conflict of interest

The author declares no conflict of interest.

Author details

Khushi Gandhi
Amity Institute of Biotechnology, Amity University, Noida, UP, India

*Address all correspondence to: khushigandhi5103@gmail.com

References

[1] Hu B, Guo H, Zhou P, Shi ZL. Characteristics of SARS-CoV-2 and COVID-19. Nature Reviews. Microbiology. 2021;**19**(3):141-154

[2] Umakanthan S, Sahu P, Ranade AV, Bukelo MM, Rao JS, Abrahao-Machado LF, et al. Origin, transmission, diagnosis and management of coronavirus disease 2019 (COVID-19). Postgraduate Medical Journal. 2020;**96**(1142):753-758

[3] World Health Organization. WHO Coronavirus (COVID-19) Dashboard [Internet] [cited 2019 Sep 9]. 2019. Available from: https://covid19.who.int/?adgroupsurvey={adgroupsurvey}&gclid=CjwKCAjwjOunBhB4EiwA94JWsLp1buk5veij5ws1d2h-DS0_O8N_ZEbVaAVVTBBxYnefjJmUseHeOBoCEiwQAvD_BwE

[4] Fernandes Q, Inchakalody VP, Merhi M, Mestiri S, Taib N, Moustafa Abo El-Ella D, et al. Emerging COVID-19 variants and their impact on SARS-CoV-2 diagnosis, therapeutics and vaccines. Annals of Medicine. 2022;**54**(1):524-540

[5] Bazargan M, Elahi R, Esmaeilzadeh A. OMICRON: Virology, immunopathogenesis, and laboratory diagnosis. The Journal of Gene Medicine. 2022;**24**(7):e3435

[6] Centers for Disease Control and Prevention. SARS-CoV-2 Variant Classifications and Definitions [Internet] [cited 2023 Sep 9]. 2019. Available from: https://www.cdc.gov/coronavirus/2019-ncov/variants/variant-classifications.html

[7] Zhang Y, Zhang H, Zhang W. SARS-CoV-2 variants, immune escape, and countermeasures. Frontiers in Medicine. 2022;**16**(2):196-207

[8] Choi JY, Smith DM. SARS-CoV-2 variants of concern. Yonsei Medical Journal. 2021;**62**(11):961

[9] Rajah MM, Hubert M, Bishop E, Saunders N, Robinot R, Grzelak L, et al. SARS-CoV-2 alpha, beta, and delta variants display enhanced spike-mediated syncytia formation. The EMBO Journal. 2021;**40**(24):e108944

[10] Magazine N, Zhang T, Wu Y, McGee MC, Veggiani G, Huang W. Mutations and evolution of the SARS-CoV-2 spike protein. Viruses. 2022;**14**(3):640

[11] McCrone JT, Hill V, Bajaj S, Pena RE, Lambert BC, Inward R, et al. Context-specific emergence and growth of the SARS-CoV-2 Delta variant. Nature. 2022;**610**(7930):154-160

[12] Zhan Y, Yin H, Yin JY. B.1.617.2 (Delta) variant of SARS-CoV-2: Features, transmission and potential strategies. International Journal of Biological Sciences. 2022;**18**(5):1844-1851

[13] Wang ML, Lin Y, Hou JF, Yang YP, Chien Y, Sun YC, et al. The Omicron variant wave: Where are we now and what are the prospects? Journal of the Chinese Medical Association. 2023;**86**(2):135-137

[14] Viana R, Moyo S, Amoako DG, Tegally H, Scheepers C, Althaus CL, et al. Rapid epidemic expansion of the SARS-CoV-2 Omicron variant in southern Africa. Nature. 2022;**603**(7902):679-686

[15] Guo Y, Han J, Zhang Y, He J, Yu W, Zhang X, et al. SARS-CoV-2 Omicron variant: Epidemiological features, biological characteristics, and clinical significance. Frontiers in Immunology. 2022;**13**:877101

[16] Rana R, Kant R, Huirem RS, Bohra D, Ganguly NK. Omicron variant: Current insights and future directions. Microbiological Research. 2022;**265**:127204

[17] Chia TRT, Young BE, Chia PY. The Omicron-transformer: Rise of the subvariants in the age of vaccines. Annals of the Academy of Medicine, Singapore. 2022;**51**(11):712-729

[18] Zhu N, Zhang D, Wang W, Li X, Yang B, Song J, et al. A novel coronavirus from patients with pneumonia in China, 2019. New England Journal of Medicine. 2020;**382**(8):727-733

[19] Wu C, Chao YW, Jiang Y, Xu HE. Structure genomics of SARS-CoV-2 and its Omicron variant: Drug design templates for COVID-19. Acta Pharmacologica Sinica. 2022;**43**(12):3021-3033

[20] Bai C, Zhong Q, Gao GF. Overview of SARS-CoV-2 genome-encoded proteins. Science China. Life Sciences. 2022;**65**(2):280-294

[21] Cao Y, Yang R, Lee I, Zhang W, Sun J, Wang W, et al. Characterization of the SARS-CoV-2 E protein: Sequence, structure, viroporin, and inhibitors. Protein Science. 2021;**30**(6):1114-1130

[22] Mohamadian M, Chiti H, Shoghli A, Biglari S, Parsamanesh N, Esmaeilzadeh A. COVID-19: Virology, biology and novel laboratory diagnosis. The Journal of Gene Medicine. 2021;**23**(2):e3303

[23] Kannan S, Shaik Syed Ali P, Sheeza A. Evolving biothreat of variant SARS-CoV-2 – molecular properties, virulence and epidemiology. European Review for Medical and Pharmacological Sciences. 2021;**25**(12):4405-4412

[24] Arya R, Kumari S, Pandey B, Mistry H, Bihani SC, Das A, et al. Structural insights into SARS-CoV-2 proteins. Journal of Molecular Biology. 2021 Jan;**433**(2):166725

[25] Tian D, Sun Y, Xu H, Ye Q. The emergence and epidemic characteristics of the highly mutated SARS-CoV-2 Omicron variant. Journal of Medical Virology. 2022;**94**(6):2376-2383

[26] Shang J, Ye G, Shi K, Wan Y, Luo C, Aihara H, et al. Structural basis of receptor recognition by SARS-CoV-2. Nature. 2020;**581**(7807):221-224

[27] Callaway E. Heavily mutated Omicron variant puts scientists on alert. Nature. 2021;**600**(7887):21-21

[28] Bayarri-Olmos R, Jarlhelt I, Johnsen LB, Hansen CB, Helgstrand C, Rose Bjelke J, et al. Functional effects of receptor-binding domain mutations of SARS-CoV-2 B.1.351 and P.1 variants. Frontiers in Immunology. 2021;**12**

[29] Wang L, Cheng G. Sequence analysis of the emerging SARS-CoV-2 variant Omicron in South Africa. Journal of Medical Virology. 2022;**94**(4):1728-1733

[30] Ford CT, Jacob Machado D, Janies DA. Predictions of the SARS-CoV-2 Omicron variant (B.1.1.529) spike protein receptor-binding domain structure and neutralizing antibody interactions. Frontiers in Virology. 2022;**2**

[31] Hoffmann M, Kleine-Weber H, Schroeder S, Krüger N, Herrler T, Erichsen S, et al. SARS-CoV-2 cell entry depends on ACE2 and TMPRSS2 and is blocked by a clinically proven protease inhibitor. Cell. 2020;**181**(2):271-280.e8

[32] Kandeel M, Mohamed MEM, Abd El-Lateef HM, Venugopala KN, El-Beltagi HS. Omicron variant genome

evolution and phylogenetics. Journal of Medical Virology. 2022;**94**(4):1627-1632

[33] Lyngse FP, Kirkeby CT, Denwood M, Christiansen LE, Mølbak K, Møller CH, et al. Household transmission of SARS-CoV-2 Omicron variant of concern subvariants BA.1 and BA.2 in Denmark. Nature Communications. 2022;**13**(1):5760

[34] Chen J, Wei GW. Omicron BA.2 (B.1.1.529.2): High potential to becoming the next dominating variant. 2022

[35] Chatterjee S, Bhattacharya M, Nag S, Dhama K, Chakraborty C. A detailed overview of SARS-CoV-2 Omicron: Its sub-variants, mutations and pathophysiology, clinical characteristics, immunological landscape, immune escape, and therapies. Viruses. 2023;**15**(1):167

[36] Lewnard JA, Hong VX, Patel MM, Kahn R, Lipsitch M, Tartof SY. Clinical outcomes associated with SARS-CoV-2 Omicron (B.1.1.529) variant and BA.1/BA.1.1 or BA.2 subvariant infection in Southern California. Nature Medicine. 2022;**28**(9):1933-1943

[37] Kawaoka Y, Uraki R, Kiso M, Iida S, Imai M, Takashita E, et al. Characterization and antiviral susceptibility of SARS-CoV-2 Omicron/BA.2. Research Sequence. 2022

[38] Yamasoba D, Kimura I, Nasser H, Morioka Y, Nao N, Ito J, et al. Virological characteristics of the SARS-CoV-2 Omicron BA.2 spike. Cell. 2022;**185**(12):2103-2115.e19

[39] Harvey WT, Carabelli AM, Jackson B, Gupta RK, Thomson EC, Harrison EM, et al. SARS-CoV-2 variants, spike mutations and immune escape. Nature Reviews. Microbiology. 2021;**19**(7):409-424

[40] Desingu PA, Nagarajan K, Dhama K. Emergence of Omicron third lineage BA.3 and its importance. Journal of Medical Virology. 2022;**94**(5):1808-1810

[41] Cao Y, Yisimayi A, Jian F, Song W, Xiao T, Wang L, et al. BA.2.12.1, BA.4 and BA.5 escape antibodies elicited by Omicron infection. Nature. 2022;**608**(7923):593-602

[42] Singhal T. The emergence of Omicron: Challenging times are Here again! Indian Journal of Pediatrics. 2022;**89**(5):490-496

[43] Grabowski F, Kochańczyk M, Lipniacki T. The spread of SARS-CoV-2 variant Omicron with a doubling time of 2.0-3.3 days can Be explained by immune evasion. Viruses. 2022;**14**(2):294

[44] Ferguson N, Ghani A, Cori A, Hogan A, Hinsley W, Volz E. Report 49: Growth, population distribution and immune escape of Omicron in England. Imperial College London. WHO Collaborating Centre for Infectious Disease Modelling, MRC Centre for Global Infectious Disease Analysis, Jameel Institute; 2021

[45] Long B, Carius BM, Chavez S, Liang SY, Brady WJ, Koyfman A, et al. Clinical update on COVID-19 for the emergency clinician: Presentation and evaluation. The American Journal of Emergency Medicine. 2022;**54**:46-57

[46] Chen J, Wang R, Gilby NB, Wei GW. Omicron variant (B.1.1.529): Infectivity, vaccine breakthrough, and antibody resistance. Journal of Chemical Information and Modeling. 2022;**62**(2):412-422

[47] Zahradník J, Marciano S, Shemesh M, Zoler E, Harari D, Chiaravalli J, et al. SARS-CoV-2 variant prediction and antiviral drug design are enabled by RBD

in vitro evolution. Nature Microbiology. 2021;**6**(9):1188-1198

[48] Hodcroft EB. CoVariants: SARS–CoV–2 Mutations and Variants of Interest [Internet] [cited 2023 Sep 9]. 2021. Available from: https://covariants.org/

[49] Shi Y, Wang Y, Shao C, Huang J, Gan J, Huang X, et al. COVID-19 infection: The perspectives on immune responses. Cell Death and Differentiation. 2020;**27**(5):1451-1454

[50] Callaway E. Are COVID surges becoming more predictable? New Omicron variants offer a hint. Nature. 2022;**605**(7909):204-206

[51] Wrapp D, Wang N, Corbett KS, Goldsmith JA, Hsieh CL, Abiona O, et al. Cryo-EM structure of the 2019-nCoV spike in the prefusion conformation. Science (1979). 2020;**367**(6483):1260-1263

[52] Pia L, Rowland-Jones S. Omicron entry route. Nature Reviews. Immunology. 2022;**22**(3):144-144

[53] Willett BJ, Grove J, MacLean OA, Wilkie C, De Lorenzo G, Furnon W, et al. SARS-CoV-2 Omicron is an immune escape variant with an altered cell entry pathway. Nature Microbiology. 2022;**7**(8):1161-1179

[54] Syed AM, Ciling A, Taha TY, Chen IP, Khalid MM, Sreekumar B, et al. Omicron mutations enhance infectivity and reduce antibody neutralization of SARS-CoV-2 virus-like particles. Proceedings of the National Academy of Sciences. 2022;**119**(31):e2200592119

[55] Peacock TP, Goldhill DH, Zhou J, Baillon L, Frise R, Swann OC, et al. The furin cleavage site in the SARS-CoV-2 spike protein is required for transmission in ferrets. Nature Microbiology. 2021;**6**(7):899-909

[56] Du X, Tang H, Gao L, Wu Z, Meng F, Yan R, et al. Omicron adopts a different strategy from Delta and other variants to adapt to host. Signal Transduction and Targeted Therapy. 2022;**7**(1):45

[57] Wolter N, Jassat W, Walaza S, Welch R, Moultrie H, Groome M, et al. Early assessment of the clinical severity of the SARS-CoV-2 Omicron variant in South Africa: A data linkage study. The Lancet. 2022;**399**(10323):437-446

[58] Mortaz E, Tabarsi P, Varahram M, Folkerts G, Adcock IM. The immune response and immunopathology of COVID-19. Frontiers in Immunology. 2020;**11**

[59] Schultze JL, Aschenbrenner AC. COVID-19 and the human innate immune system. Cell. 2021;**184**(7):1671-1692

[60] Valizadeh H, Abdolmohammadi-vahid S, Danshina S, Ziya Gencer M, Ammari A, Sadeghi A, et al. Nano-curcumin therapy, a promising method in modulating inflammatory cytokines in COVID-19 patients. International Immunopharmacology. 2020;**89**:107088

[61] Azkur AK, Akdis M, Azkur D, Sokolowska M, van de Veen W, Brüggen M, et al. Immune response to SARS-CoV-2 and mechanisms of immunopathological changes in COVID-19. Allergy. 2020;**75**(7):1564-1581

[62] Cao Y, Su B, Guo X, Sun W, Deng Y, Bao L, et al. Potent neutralizing antibodies against SARS-CoV-2 identified by high-throughput single-cell sequencing of convalescent patients' B cells. Cell. 2020;**182**(1):73-84.e16

[63] Ju B, Zhang Q, Ge J, Wang R, Sun J, Ge X, et al. Human neutralizing antibodies elicited by SARS-CoV-2 infection. Nature. 2020;**584**(7819):115-119

[64] Kared H, Wolf AS, Alirezaylavasani A, Ravussin A, Solum G, Tran TT, et al. Immune responses in Omicron SARS-CoV-2 breakthrough infection in vaccinated adults. Nature Communications. 2022;**13**(1):4165

[65] Kupferschmidt K, Vogel G. How bad is Omicron? Some clues are emerging. Science (1979). 2021;**374**(6573):1304-1305

[66] Chen N, Zhou M, Dong X, Qu J, Gong F, Han Y, et al. Epidemiological and clinical characteristics of 99 cases of 2019 novel coronavirus pneumonia in Wuhan, China: A descriptive study. The Lancet. 2020;**395**(10223):507-513

[67] Zheng YY, Ma YT, Zhang JY, Xie X. COVID-19 and the cardiovascular system. Nature Reviews. Cardiology. 2020;**17**(5):259-260

[68] Menni C, Valdes AM, Polidori L, Antonelli M, Penamakuri S, Nogal A, et al. Symptom prevalence, duration, and risk of hospital admission in individuals infected with SARS-CoV-2 during periods of Omicron and delta variant dominance: A prospective observational study from the ZOE COVID study. The Lancet. 2022;**399**(10335):1618-1624

[69] Garrett N, Tapley A, Andriesen J, Seocharan I, Fisher LH, Bunts L, et al. High rate of asymptomatic carriage associated with variant strain Omicron. medRxiv. 2022;**399**:1618-1624

[70] Halfmann PJ, Iida S, Iwatsuki-Horimoto K, Maemura T, Kiso M, Scheaffer SM, et al. SARS-CoV-2 Omicron virus causes attenuated disease in mice and hamsters. Nature. 2022;**603**(7902):687-692

[71] Gandhi K, Khare S, Sachdeva R. Significance of biochemical and hematological indicators in predicting COVID-19 prognosis during the Omicron variant phase – A retrospective study. Medicine India. 2022;**1**:11

[72] Suzuki R, Yamasoba D, Kimura I, Wang L, Kishimoto M, Ito J, et al. Attenuated fusogenicity and pathogenicity of SARS-CoV-2 Omicron variant. Nature. 2022;**603**(7902):700-705

[73] Shuai H, Chan JFW, Hu B, Chai Y, Yuen TTT, Yin F, et al. Attenuated replication and pathogenicity of SARS-CoV-2 B.1.1.529 Omicron. Nature. 2022;**603**(7902):693-699

[74] Bouzid D, Visseaux B, Kassasseya C, Daoud A, Fémy F, Hermand C, et al. Comparison of patients infected with delta versus Omicron COVID-19 variants presenting to Paris emergency departments. Annals of Internal Medicine. 2022;**175**(6):831-837

[75] Feikin DR, Abu-Raddad LJ, Andrews N, Davies MA, Higdon MM, Orenstein WA, et al. Assessing vaccine effectiveness against severe COVID-19 disease caused by Omicron variant. Report from a meeting of the World Health Organization. Vaccine. 2022;**40**(26):3516-3527

[76] Chen X, Yan X, Sun K, Zheng N, Sun R, Zhou J, et al. Estimation of disease burden and clinical severity of COVID-19 caused by Omicron BA.2 in Shanghai, February-June 2022. Emerging Microbes and Infection. 2022;**11**(1):2800-2807

[77] Esmaeilzadeh A, Elahi R. Immunobiology and immunotherapy of COVID-19: A clinically updated overview. Journal of Cellular Physiology. 2021;**236**(4):2519-2543

[78] Liu J, Li S, Liu J, Liang B, Wang X, Wang H, et al. Longitudinal characteristics of lymphocyte responses and cytokine profiles in the peripheral blood of SARS-CoV-2 infected patients. eBioMedicine. 2020;**55**:102763

[79] Esmaeilzadeh A, Jafari D, Tahmasebi S, Elahi R, Khosh E. Immune-based therapy for COVID-19. 2021; 449-468.

[80] Elahi R, Karami P, Heidary AH, Esmaeilzadeh A. An updated overview of recent advances, challenges, and clinical considerations of IL-6 signaling blockade in severe coronavirus disease 2019 (COVID-19). International Immunopharmacology. 2022;**105**:108536

[81] Hojyo S, Uchida M, Tanaka K, Hasebe R, Tanaka Y, Murakami M, et al. How COVID-19 induces cytokine storm with high mortality. Inflammation Regeneration. 2020;**40**(1):37

[82] Esmaeilzadeh A, Rostami S, Yeganeh PM, Tahmasebi S, Ahmadi M. Recent advances in antibody-based immunotherapy strategies for COVID-19. Journal of Cellular Biochemistry. 2021;**122**(10):1389-1412

[83] Batah SS, Fabro AT. Pulmonary pathology of ARDS in COVID-19: A pathological review for clinicians. Respiratory Medicine. 2021;**176**:106239

[84] Wilhelm A, Widera M, Grikscheit K, Toptan T, Schenk B, Pallas C, et al. Limited neutralisation of the SARS-CoV-2 Omicron subvariants BA.1 and BA.2 by convalescent and vaccine serum and monoclonal antibodies. eBioMedicine. 2022;**82**:104158

[85] Cele S, Jackson L, Khoury DS, Khan K, Moyo-Gwete T, Tegally H, et al. SARS-CoV-2 Omicron has extensive but incomplete escape of Pfizer BNT162b2 elicited neutralization and requires ACE2 for infection. medRxiv. 2021;**176**:106239

[86] Guihot A, Litvinova E, Autran B, Debré P, Vieillard V. Cell-mediated immune responses to COVID-19 infection. Frontiers in Immunology. 2020;**82**:104158

[87] Iqbal H. The importance of cell-mediated immunity in COVID-19 – An opinion. Medical Hypotheses. 2020;**143**:110152

[88] Boechat JL, Chora I, Morais A, Delgado L. The immune response to SARS-CoV-2 and COVID-19 immunopathology – Current perspectives. Pulmonology. 2021;**27**(5):423-437

[89] Gowrisankar A, Priyanka TMC, Banerjee S. Omicron: A mysterious variant of concern. The European Physical Journal Plus. 2022;**137**(1):100

[90] Li C, Zhao C, Bao J, Tang B, Wang Y, Gu B. Laboratory diagnosis of coronavirus disease-2019 (COVID-19). Clinica Chimica Acta. 2020;**510**:35-46

[91] Tahmasebi S, Khosh E, Esmaeilzadeh A. The outlook for diagnostic purposes of the 2019-novel coronavirus disease. Journal of Cellular Physiology. 2020;**235**(12):9211-9229

[92] Ettaboina SK, Nakkala K, Laddha KS. A mini review on SARS-COVID-19-2 Omicron variant (B.1.1.529). SciMed Journal. 2021;**3**(4):399-406

[93] Chen X, Kang Y, Luo J, Pang K, Xu X, Wu J, et al. Next-generation sequencing reveals the progression of COVID-19. Frontiers in Cellular and Infection Microbiology. 2021;**11**:11

[94] Allam M, Ismail A, Khumalo ZTH, Kwenda S, van Heusden P, Cloete R, et al. Genome sequencing of a severe acute respiratory syndrome coronavirus 2 isolate obtained from a south African patient with coronavirus disease 2019. Microbiology Resources Announcement. 2020;**9**(27):632490

[95] Li D, Li J. Immunologic testing for SARS-CoV-2 infection from the antigen perspective. Journal of Clinical Microbiology. 2021;**59**(5):e00572-e00620

[96] Yuan M, Liu H, Wu NC, Wilson IA. Recognition of the SARS-CoV-2 receptor binding domain by neutralizing antibodies. Biochemical and Biophysical Research Communications. 2021;**538**:192-203

[97] Hurt AC, Wheatley AK. Neutralizing antibody therapeutics for COVID-19. Viruses. 2021;**13**(4):628

[98] Cameroni E, Saliba C, Bowen JE, Rosen LE, Culap K, Pinto D, et al. Broadly neutralizing antibodies overcome SARS-CoV-2 Omicron antigenic shift. bioRxiv. 2021;**538**:192-203

[99] Tao K, Tzou PL, Kosakovsky Pond SL, Ioannidis JPA, Shafer RW. Susceptibility of SARS-CoV-2 Omicron variants to therapeutic monoclonal antibodies: Systematic review and meta-analysis. Microbiology Spectroscopy. 2022;**10**(4):628

[100] Zhou H, Møhlenberg M, Thakor JC, Tuli HS, Wang P, Assaraf YG, et al. Sensitivity to vaccines, therapeutic antibodies, and viral entry inhibitors and advances to counter the SARS-CoV-2 Omicron variant. Nature. Dec 2022;**602**:664-670

[101] Garcia-Beltran WF, Denis KJ, Hoelzemer A, Lam EC, Nitido AD, Sheehan ML, et al. mRNA-based COVID-19 vaccine boosters induce neutralizing immunity against SARS-CoV-2 Omicron variant. Cell. 2022;**185**(3):457-466.e4

[102] Shrestha LB, Foster C, Rawlinson W, Tedla N, Bull RA. Evolution of the SARS-CoV-2 Omicron variants BA.1 to BA.5: Implications for immune escape and transmission. Reviews in Medical Virology. 2022;**32**(5):e0001422

[103] Zhang L, Cao L, Gao XS, Zheng BY, Deng YQ, Li JX, et al. A proof of concept for neutralizing antibody-guided vaccine design against SARS-CoV-2. National Science Review. 2021;**185**:457-466.e4

[104] Sun C, Kang YF, Liu YT, Kong XW, Xu HQ, Xiong D, et al. Parallel profiling of antigenicity alteration and immune escape of SARS-CoV-2 Omicron and other variants. Signal Transduction and Targeted Therapy. 2022;**7**(1):42

[105] Cerutti G, Guo Y, Liu L, Liu L, Zhang Z, Luo Y, et al. Cryo-EM structure of the SARS-CoV-2 Omicron spike. Cell Reports. 2022;**38**(9):110428

[106] U.S. National Library of Medicine. ClincalTrial.gov [Internet]. [cited 2023 Sep 10]. 2023. Available from: https://classic.clinicaltrials.gov/ct2/results?term=vaccine&cond=Omicron&recrs=d&age_v=&gndr=&type=&rslt=&phase=2&phase=3&Search=Apply

Chapter 3

Production and Formation of SARS-CoV-2 Variants

Ishrat Perveen, Bakhtawar Bukhari, Naaz Abbas, Sania Mazhar, Yasar Saleem, Shaista Nawaz, Samia Nawab, Quratulain Syed, Syed Hussain Imam Abidi, Sana Riaz, Ramsha Essa, Abad Ali Nadeem, Muhammad Farooq, Fatima Akram and Saba Sabahat

Abstract

The emergence of severe acute respiratory syndrome coronavirus 2 (SARS-CoV-2) variants has been considered responsible for the prolonged continuation of the coronavirus disease 2019 (COVID-19) pandemic. The fast dissemination of these variants presents a challenge for current vaccines. Next-generation vaccinations must be manufactured and distributed quickly to stop the pandemic. To combat existing variations and stop the development of new ones, coordinated surveillance, the designing of new vaccines, and broad-scale immunization are required. Clinical trials are still being conducted to assess the efficacy of the vaccination against various SARS-CoV-2 variants.

Keywords: mutant, variants, serology, omicron, SARS-CoV-2, COVID-19

1. Introduction

Since its emergence, coronavirus disease 2019 (COVID-19) has resulted in 520,912,257 and 6,272,408 confirmed cases and deaths, respectively. Scientists have been reported to produce a variety of vaccines, with 198 in preliminary stages of development and 156 in worldwide clinical trials. There have been 11,713,606,779 doses of vaccine provided since May 16, 2022. The total number of confirmed infections has dramatically grown after October 11, 2021, yet there has not been a discernible change in the COVID-19 incidence since that date. As a result, there is now a greater chance of developing new mutations, such as variants of concern (VOC) and variants of interest (VOI), which have a greater potential of spreading and infecting others while being less likely to be recognized by host antibodies. This chapter will keep track of the most recent SARS-CoV-2 variations and mutations, provide an overview of therapeutic studies, and discuss current pandemic-fighting issues and potential solutions.

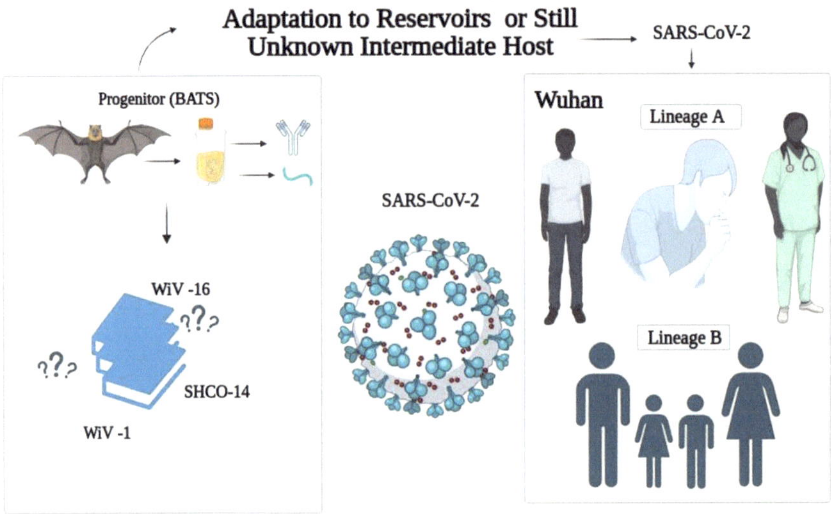

Figure 1.
Natural origin of SARSCoV2 lineages.

2. Origin of SARS-CoV-2

Severe acute respiratory syndrome coronavirus 2 (SARSCoV2) shares approximately eighty percent (79%) homology with SARS-CoV, and other highly deadly human coronaviruses have been zoonotic in origin. A significant quantity of antibodies against SARS-CoV-2 were discovered in isolates of the virus of Himalayan palm tree civets and raccoon dogs. Bats serve as a major reservoir for several SARS-like viruses due to their infection with SARS-CoV-2 and other ancestors of the SARS virus. Horseshoe bats that had taken up residence in caverns in the Yunan region of mainland China were found as the first reservoir for the emergence of SARS-CoV-2. The distance in time and space between the ancient Yunnan caves and the initial appearance of SARS-CoV-2, however, emphasizes how challenging it is to find out the virus transmission pathways. SARS-CoV-2 originated in China in 2019, disseminated through dense populations of live animals that may have been infected with SARS-CoV2, and is now globally transmitted through human-to-human transmission, with higher susceptibility in carnivores such as cats, ferrets, and raccoon dogs. Further investigation is needed to determine its potential in animal populations. The natural origin of SARS-CoV-2 lineages is depicted in **Figure 1**.

3. SARS-CoV-2 and evolutionary lineages

A ribonucleic acid (RNA) virus called SARS-CoV-2 possesses a 3-to-5 exonuclease enabling high-fidelity reproduction. As a consequence of the COVID-19 pandemic, nearly three thousand (2920) genomes were collected between December 2019 and April 2022, and these variants of the SARS-CoV-2 virus are unique. These genetic lineages have been identified and followed using Nextstrain, Pango, and the Global Initiative on Sharing All Influenza Data (GISAID). The World Health Organization (WHO) has named two VOIs and VOCs using Greek alphabet letters to prevent confusion.

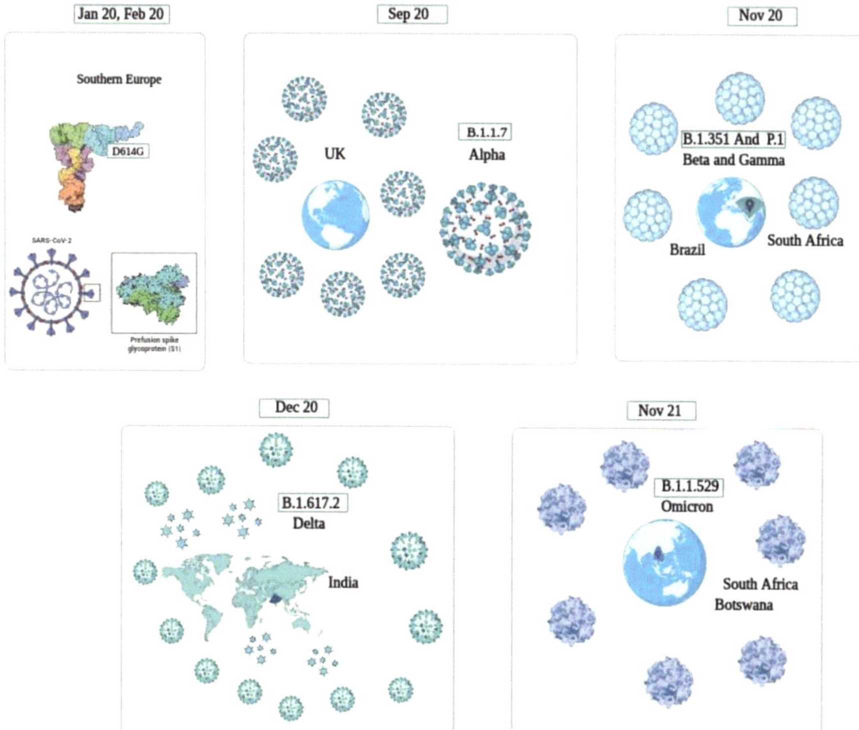

Figure 2.
Emergence of SARS-CoV-2 variants.

Despite mutations, it replicates efficiently, with an evolution rate of 2 mutations per month between 2019 and 2020. The 614G variant of SARS-CoV-2 has gained global attention due to its superior viral entry and replication efficiency and its higher fitness compared to the 614D variant. Consequently, variants of concern (VOC) have emerged.

The ecological behavior of SARS-CoV-2 emphasizes the potential for cross-species transmission, evident in cases involving farmed minks, dogs, cats, and lions in zoos. When animals are infected, the virus has the opportunity to evolve and adapt, as observed in minks in the Netherlands and Denmark. Infections in animals carrying the human SARS-CoV-2 strain might lead to recombination events, potentially giving rise to hybrid viruses with pandemic potential. The newly discovered VOCs and VOIs of SARS-CoV-2 have been reported to indicate worse clinical symptoms, higher transmissibility, diagnostic detection challenges, escape from vaccine-induced or innate immunity, and adverse therapeutic responses. The most important variants are Alpha, Beta, and Gamma. The Delta variant's frequency increased rapidly, with Omicron currently accounting for 5% [1]. Detailed information regarding the dates and countries of emergence of SARS-CoV-2 variants have been depicted in **Figure 2**.

4. SARS-CoV-2 variants and their characteristics

Current COVID-19 vaccines elicit broad immune responses, protecting new virus variants such as Omicron; more research is needed to determine their effectiveness.

Variants are divided into several classes by the WHO and the Center for Disease Control and Prevention (CDC). A SARS-CoV-2's VOI differs from earlier strains of the virus in that it has alterations that are possibly to blame for the virus's enhanced transmissibility and the capacity to elude diagnostic tests, evade immunity, or cause severe illnesses. A VOC is potentially transmissible and more likely to induce new infections. This category includes the delta and omicron versions. A high-impact variant is one from which current immunizations do not offer protection. There are no any SARS-CoV-2 variants in this category right now. The WHO classified VOCs of SARS-CoV-2 with enhanced virulence, transmissibility, and resistance to current therapeutic vaccines, diagnostics, and other such medical techniques. Notable VOCs include alpha (α), beta (β), gamma (γ), delta (δ), and omicron. The SARS-CoV-2 life-cycle begins with the S1 receptor-binding domain (RBD) and angiotensin-converting enzyme 2 (ACE2) interacting, causing the S protein to divide into S2 subunits. The S protein is degraded by the furin that further triggers the virus particles to enter the cellular membrane of the host cell. Sixteen nonstructural proteins are produced, which are followed by their translation into replicase protein and their destruction by proteases. Double-membrane vesicles (DMVs) aid in RNA replication, whereas E, M, and S proteins create mature virions for infection. The mechanism of SARS-CoV-2 infection is depicted in **Figure 3**.

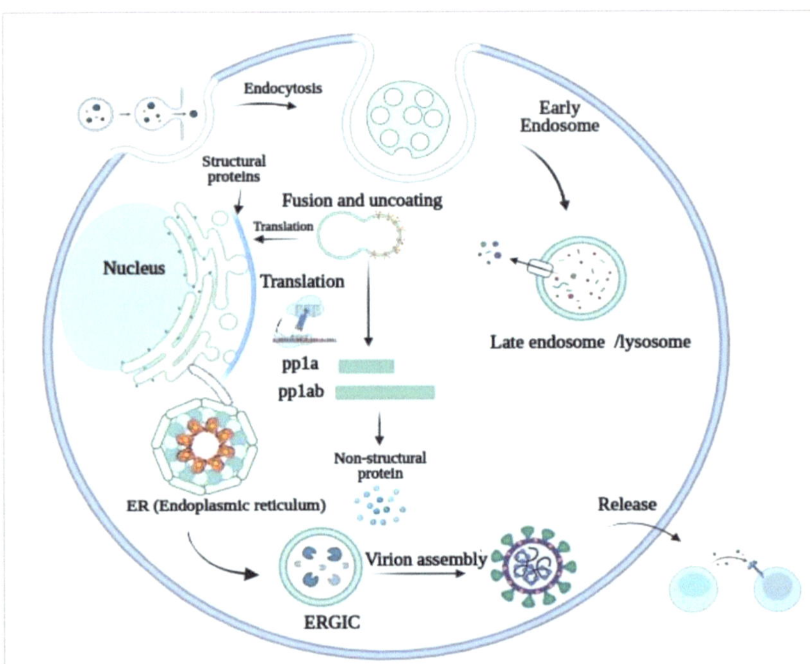

Figure 3.
*Mechanistic pathway of SARS-CoV-2 infection: The replication process of SARS-CoV-2 involves the development of DMVs (double-membrane vesicles) in host cells. Viral RNAs are retained in DMVs and transferred for assembly or translation to the cytosol. Structural proteins form viral particles, whereas sgRNAs encode auxiliary proteins. N protein and RNA synthesis occur in the cytoplasm, whereas E, M, and S proteins are produced in the ER (endoplasmic reticulum). Two thirds of the genome's replicase genes are translated into two big polyproteins, pp1a and pp1ab, and from there, sixteen types of nonstructural proteins (NSP) are produced. The viral RNA-N complex, E, M, and S proteins then enter the ERGIC, where mature virions are assembled. The ERGIC further undergoes significant N-glycosylation, controlling protein folding, stability, infectiousness, and immunological evasion [2]. *pp1a, pp1ab: Large polyproteins; ERGIC: Endoplasmic reticulum-Golgi intermediate compartment.*

The initial stage in replication is the development of DMVs (vesicles with double membranes) in a host cell brought by the COVID-19 infection. NSP3 and NSP4 stimulate the replication of both sgRNA (subgenomic RNA) and gRNAs (genomic RNAs) and cause the endoplasmic reticulum's (ER) reorganization into DMV [3]. The viral RNAs are retained in DMVs and either transferred via double-membrane-spanning pores for the viral assembly or to the cytosol for translation [4]. Structural proteins assemble gRNA into viral particles, whereas sgRNAs encode auxiliary and conserved structural proteins. RNA and N protein synthesis takes place in the cytoplasm, whereas S, M, and E proteins are produced in the endoplasmic reticulum, or ER, and transported to the Golgi system. The SARS-CoV-2 genome consists of replicase genes translated into pp1a and pp1ab polyproteins, processed into 16 NSPs, and assembled in the ERGIC compartment. These virions then escape the Golgi apparatus and cell membrane. In the ERGIC, the S protein monomer undergoes substantial N-glycosylation modification as well. In addition to controlling protein folding, glycosylation of virus proteins additionally influences virus stability, infectiousness, and immunological evasion (**Figure 3**). Studies have discovered 26 mutations, which tend to include six of interest (K417T, N501Y, P681H, L452R, and L18F), with a prevalence rate of more than 75% in at least one lineage across VOCs (five) and VOIs (two). These mutations were found in at least 20% of countries, with N501Y, E484Q, K417N, T478K, S477N, L452R, and E484Q associated with increased ACE2 binding.

4.1 Alpha (α-variant lineage-B.1.1.7)

In 2020 and 2021, three variant strains B.1.351, P.1 COVs, and B.1.1.7, first appeared in the UK (United Kingdom), South Africa, and Brazil. Increased transmission and decreased neutralization that may tend to have an impact on monoclonal antibodies are well-known characteristics of the alpha and beta versions. Mortality and hospitalization to the intensive care unit have risen with alpha variants. Alpha is significantly protected against by the BNT162b2 vaccine; however, the mRNA-1273 vaccine exhibits less neutralization. Gamma variations are less susceptible to therapies and past vaccines and convalescent-serum neutralization.

B.1.1.7, first discovered in September 2020 in the UK and later in the US, has 17 mutations in its genome. Notably, there were eight mutations in the spike protein of the Alpha version, including the deletion of D1118H, N501Y, T716I, A570D, P681H, S982A, D144, and D69–70. The B.1.1.7 protein undergoes amino acid changes that improve ACE2 affinity and RBD accessibility, which may become the reason for enhanced transmissibility.

The protein SARS-CoV2-S is destabilized by the N501Y mutation, which also increases RBD-ACE2 affinity and accelerates the propagation of SARS-CoV-2. Additionally, compared to those infected with other variations, those exposed to the variant lineages of B.1.1.7 suffered from a considerably severe illness and had a greater risk of dying.

4.2 Beta (β- variant lineage 20H and/or B.1.351)

Beta variant has been found responsible for the emergence of the second wave of COVID-19 in the Bay of Nelson Mandela. It was discovered in South Africa (SA) by the end of 2020 [5].

The β-form of the spike protein has nine mutations, which include L18F, N501Y, R246I, E484K, D215G, K417N, A701V, D614G, and D80A. It has been reported that there have been three changes made to the receptor binding domain (RBD) to enhance receptor affinity.

The E484K mutation alters antibody binding to the receptor-binding domain, whereas the N501Y substitution is found in fast-expanding lineages. These mutations play critical roles in disease transmission and outbreaks, increasing compatibility towards human ACE2, and their combination enhances this attraction.

The Beta variant of SARS-CoV-2 has a unique amino acid alteration, P71L, in its E protein, linked to illness severity and death rate, but its impact remains uncertain. It may have a selective advantage.

4.3 Gamma (γ-P.1 lineage)

Eleven mutations in spike protein and three mutations in the region of the receptor-binding domain resulted in the emergence of γ -P.1 variant lineage, which was initially discovered in January 2021 in the United States of America (USA) [6].

Eleven mutations, including L18F, R190S, T1027I, N501Y, K417T, and E484K, D138Y, P26S, H655Y, V1176, and T20N, have been found in the variant's spike protein. In addition, three changes (K417N, L18F, and E484K) in the RBD of the Gamma (γ) version are comparable to those in the Beta (β) variant.

4.4 Delta (δ-variant lineage B.1.617.2)

Since its discovery in India in 2020, the Delta (-B.1.617.2) mutant lineage has quickly expanded and boosted transmissibility in homes and indoor sports. Additionally, it lessens the neutralization of monoclonal emergency use authorization (EUA) antibody therapies. The efficiency of the Delta vaccine is just 33%, whereas the efficacy of the ChAdOx1 and BNT162b2 nCoV-19 vaccines after two doses is still more than 67%. In April 2021, it was discovered that it had a major effect on the COVID-19 pandemic's second wave. The Delta variety, which was discovered for the first time in the United States (US) in March 2021, is extremely contagious and prevalent in many nations. It has 11 mutations in the spike protein. It possesses eleven mutations in the protein known as spike [6].

4.5 Omicron (SARS-CoV-2 variant lineage B.1.1.529)

The latest SARS-CoV-2 variant, VOC "Omicron" was first reported in November 2021 in the South Africa (SA) region. This variant has exhibited 50 mutations, thirty-two of which were targeting spike protein and three of which affect the cleavage site of furin and so increase infectivity. The lineage B.1.1.529VOC variant is considered the most contagious form identified and may resist immune defenses provided by current vaccinations or prior infections. According to GISAID, the virus had 6950 cases and had spread to 86 nations and territories by December 16, 2021. Recent research revealed that following immunization with the Pfizer-BioNTech (BNT162b2) vaccine, serum's neutralization activity against the Omicron variation was forty-one (41.4) times below the original strain; however, the escape was only partially successful. The Omicron variant has a significant capacity to overcome previous infection-related immunity (Ferré et al., 2022).

Since its discovery in November 2021 in South Africa, the Omicron variety has been found in more than 100 nations and areas worldwide. The WHO classified it as a VOC and categorized it among those variants under monitoring. Omicron has 50 mutations,

DOI: http://dx.doi.org/10.5772/intechopen.1003717

30 on the surface S protein, 20 novels in the S1 domain, eight in neglected tropical diseases (NTDs), and 15 in RBD. These modifications may improve RBD-ACE2 interaction and accelerate transmission. Omicron's 3-day incubation time and cold-like symptoms are attributed to its insertion sequence. Omicron, unlike typical influenza, exhibits distinct symptoms such as smell and taste loss, persists in the body, and can reactivate, potentially leading to fatalities. The CDC detected the omicron virus in New York City's wastewater 10 days before the US first reported illness and South Africa confirmed its presence. Researchers in California, Texas, and France also identified variants. The discovery of omicron presence in certain areas during a specific period holds significant implications for the detection and spread of the virus [7].

4.6 Lambda (λ- C.37 variant lineage) and mu (μ- B.1.621 variant lineage)

The WHO has identified two variants as Lambda (λ) and Mu (μ) lineage variants. The L452Q mutation within RBD of the spike protein, which was initially found in C.37 in Peru and Chile in 2020, improves the virus's virulence, transmissibility, and infectivity. Recent research demonstrates lower susceptibility to neutralization by convalescent sera and the monoclonal antibody REGN10987 as well as a three (3.05) time reduction in neutralization as compared to the wild-type virus. When compared to the WA1 strain, B.1.621, which was discovered for the first time in January 2021 in Colombia, had a 2.3-fold lower neutralizing antibody response.

5. Major physiological differences among mutant strains

There are now 4 SARS-CoV-2's VOCs, that is, α- (B.1.1.7), β- (B.1.351), γ - (P.1), and (δ) delta (B.1.617.2). They have shown D614G mutation, which confers higher infectivity, most likely because of alterations in receptor binding or fusion. The N501Y mutation is carried out by α, β, and γ, boosting their receptor-binding efficacy and cellular entrance. Fortunately, combining mutations may result in more conformational alterations and different alterations. VOCs, for example, have varying receptor-binding sites. Separation from the receptor requires the most effort, followed by β/γ or delta.

5.1 Plaque sizes

In Vero E6 cells, all these variations had a distinct plaque size. Beta had the greatest mean plaque size, next to gamma, delta, and alpha. In Vero E6 Transmembrane Protease, Serine2 (TMPRSS2) cells, a comparable result with varied plaque diameters was found. There are various variables of plaque size, including receptor-binding affinities heat stability and viral reproduction rate. If a variation is more stable at physiological temperatures and produces more offspring viruses, it creates larger infectious viral particles, attacking a greater number of cells and raising plaque size.

5.2 Thermal stability

The beta version is the most stable of the 4 VOCs at 4, 24, and 37°C. With a half-life nearly double that of γ or delta, β has the strongest thermal stability. Except for alpha, there is a link between heat stability and plaque size. Interestingly, despite its small plaque size, alpha has a relatively extended half-life, implying an alternate process.

5.3 Viral replication rates

Although there are no substantial changes in viral RNA replica number, Alpha has fewer pathogenic particles than the other versions. Furthermore, alpha and gamma intracellular viral RNA concentrations are substantially lower than those of the other VOCs. Alpha's viral replication rate is probably inadequate, which contributes to its limited plaque size [8].

6. How to control novel varieties and recurrent outbreaks?

Controlling the pandemic is challenging because of recurrent outbreaks and novel varieties. Effective vaccinations and antiviral therapies are crucial in the early stages, but anti-inflammatory and immunomodulatory therapy could be more effective in later stages. SARS-CoV-2 infection suppression requires monoclonal antibodies, nanobodies, recovered plasma, mini proteins, soluble ACE2, and receptor ACE2 traps, targeting host proteases like furin and TMPRSS2 [9]. The development of a disease is greatly influenced by immune responses, and the SARS-CoV-2 evasion pathways are still poorly known. Immunomodulators have antiviral effects, but their effectiveness in treating COVID-19 remains uncertain. Traditional Chinese medicine effectively combats viruses through immune modulation, whereas vaccine development involves selecting antigens, enhancing sequences, screening nucleotides, evaluating the immune response, and conducting safety tests, with RNA vaccines being the most effective [10]. The mechanistic pathways indicating various mechanisms of antiviral CoV19 therapeutics by inhibiting SARS-CoV-2 entrance, preventing SARS-CoV-2 replication, application of immunomodulators, and vaccine development have been shown in **Figure 4**.

Inhibiting the initial stages (*i.e.*, attachment and penetration) of SARS-COV-2 infection is crucial for disease prevention. Primary S protein inhibitors include human soluble ACE2, ACE2 receptor trap compounds, nanobodies, miniproteins, convalescent plasma, and monoclonal antibodies [11]. Coreceptors, which block SARS-CoV-2 infection, have been identified as potential therapeutic targets for COVID-19 treatment, with inhibitors and generic particles potentially reducing infection (**Figure 4A**). SARS-CoV-2 enters host cells through endosomal or receptor-mediated membrane fusion, requiring protease inhibitors like furin and TMMPRS2 to prevent fusion entrance. SARS-COV-2 infection has been demonstrated to be reduced to variable degrees by both TMPRSS2 and furin inhibitors (**Figure 4A**).

Antiviral therapy uses blocking viral proteins and RNA synthesis to reduce viral replication. Mpro and PLpro, proteases crucial for viral replication, have potential therapeutic targets. Mpro inhibitors are now in various phases of preclinical and clinical research (**Figure 4B**) [12]. The immune system's role in SARS-COV-2 evasion is not fully understood, and the therapeutic benefits of immunomodulators such as ivermectin and interferon on COVID-19 are debatable. The first CoV19 antibody developed by China fetched international approval in December 2021. It has been given commercial approval under the name BRII-196/BRII-198 (**Figure 4C**) [13, 14].

There are currently almost 340 vaccines widely available against the SARS-CoV-2. One hundred and twenty-two are being applied in various clinical trials. Thirty vaccines, however, are regularly being used worldwide. Primary types include inactivated, attenuated live, DNA/RNA, vector-based, and unidentified forms.

DOI: http://dx.doi.org/10.5772/intechopen.1003717

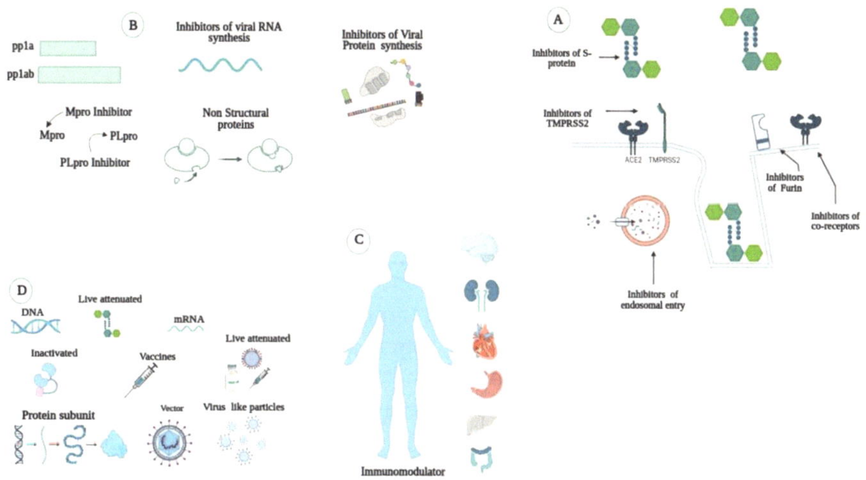

Figure 4.
*Antiviral CoV19 therapeutics. A) Inhibition of SARSCoV2 entrance, B) inhibition of SARSCoV2 replication, C) Immunomodulators, and D) vaccine development. * pp1a, pp1ab: Large polyproteins; Mpro:Main protease inhibitor; Plpro:Papain-like protease.*

RNA vaccines are the most effective vaccines worldwide (**Figure 4D**) [15, 16]. Future vaccines are expected to offer protection against both current and upcoming SARS-CoV-2 variant strains.

7. COVID-19 vaccine effectiveness on SARS-CoV-2 variants

COVID-19 precise inoculations sanctioned under EUA are distributed into four kinds: inactivated, viral vector, nucleic acid, and subunit. These vaccines rely on the SARS-CoV-2's S protein to induce neutralizing antibodies. However, the advent of SARS-CoV-2 variants led to hurdles in vaccine improvement. Mutations on the spike protein resulted in improved transmission, severe ailment, diminished neutralization, and invulnerable invasion. VOCs are highly contagious and are related to greater hospitalization rates and death.

7.1 Alpha variant and clinical vaccine trials

The vaccine ChAdOx1, tested against α-variant, showed lower neutralization activity in contradiction to non-Alpha variants. Defensive efficiencies against Alpha (α) and non-Alpha variants were reportedly found at 70% and 81%, respectively. The NVX-CoV2373 vaccine, which was tested contrary to the Alpha variant, exhibited an efficiency of 86.30% in contrast to α variants and 96.40% against non-Alpha variants. The vaccine also showed a 51.0% efficiency in contrast to the β variant. Both vaccines showed acceptable protection against α variant and non-Alpha variants, but their effectiveness must be assessed in a greater population. Additional investigation is required to assess the immunogenicity, efficacy, and shelter of these vaccines [17].

7.2 Beta variant and clinical vaccine trials

The vaccine ChAdOx1-nCoV-19 was invented by AstraZeneca followed by the approval from the University of Oxford to check COVID-19 in adults. A South African trial found that the inoculation's effectiveness against the β-variant was 10.40%, indicating a substandard shield against mild to moderate COVID-19 triggered by β variant. The Ad26.COV2.S vaccine, a nonreplicating human adenovirus type 26 vector, was accepted for checking COVID-19 in persons over teenage years under EUA. A Phase 3 study assessed the usefulness and protection of this vaccine for the preclusion of β-variant in adults aged above 18 years. In animal prototypes, the NVX-CoV2373 vaccine, which contains Matrix-M1 adjuvant, and the full-length of SARS-CoV-2's spike protein has shown adequate security, robust neutralizing antibodies, and cellular immune reactivity. However, the efficiency of this inoculation in a situation of continuing β variant transmission is immediately assessed.

7.3 Delta variant and clinical vaccine trials

The Delta variant of COVID-19 has become the dominant variant due to its enlarged transmissibility in indoor game locations. Studies show that neutralizing antibody titers decrease after BNT162b2 vaccination against Delta and β variants compared to α variants. However, larger sample sizes are needed for verification. A Phase 3 randomized, placebo-controlled, double-blind therapeutic trial in India evaluated the efficacy of BBV152 vaccination against the Delta variant, achieving a 65.2% success rate [18].

8. Current challenges of combating SARS-CoV-2's VOCs

The COVID-19 outbreak has been a notable global health emergency, and management has become more difficult as a result of the development and rapid spread of variations of concern (VOCs). VOCs may be more suitable because they are antigenically different from the original SARS-associated viruses that caused the first outbreak of the disease and looked to be able to reinfect humans more successfully. The epidemic, which also caused social and economic problems, caused millions of deaths. There are concerns that the emergence and propagation of novel strains of infections might indicate that our global struggle against the pandemic may need to extend much longer than planned. The next great health disaster to impact society may be COVID-19.

It is noteworthy that COVID-19 immunizations were approved in less than a year, both in human history and in the area of medicine. Numerous obstacles still exist, including the need for storage, transportation, and the universal provision of vaccinations to more than 7 billion people. In other countries, the lack of vaccines and slow supplies make it more difficult to contain the pandemic and may encourage the creation of novel varieties that might lengthen the spread of the disease.

VOCs reduce the analytical techniques' RT-PCR-based identification sensitivity, which results in false-negative detection. Vaccine hesitancy, an increasing worry, may thwart efforts to combat the virus and boost societal confidence, particularly in underserved communities. Because of their increased virulence and transmission, the recently discovered SARS-CoV-2 VOCs provide new, global approaches to controlling this epidemic. COVID-19 vaccines are manufactured using a variety of machines and stages that target spike protein and receptor-binding characteristics. Efficacy ranges from 65–95%, with RNA vaccines having an efficacy as high as 95%. The aforementioned vaccines require two administrations with a gap of 20–30 days to be effective to provide protection. However, because the virus is constantly changing, recently created vaccinations seem to be ineffective. It is crucial to monitor the emergence of the SARS-associated animal species considering the uncertainty of total eradication. The current vaccination campaign may not provide complete protection to all individuals or subpopulations, leaving certain areas susceptible. The virus may persist due to ongoing risks of infection and the potential for additional dispersion among vulnerable human hosts.

9. Pragmatic future strategies

The widespread distribution of VOCs, which have enhanced transmission and impeded the effectiveness of vaccinations and monoclonal antibodies, has worsened the current SARS-CoV-2 epidemic. Strategies include preserving public separation, proper sanitation, and mask use are essential to lowering morbidity and death. Nonpharmaceutical interventions (*i.e.,* NPIs) are another important strategy. Because of the ineffectiveness or inaccessibility of VOC vaccinations, these techniques aid in containing current outbreaks and preventing future ones.

As virus duplication suggests multiple experimental COVID-19 demonstrations, antiviral medication is advised for treating mild to moderate SARS-CoV-2 disease. Antiviral medications such as ivermectin, hydroxychloroquine, nitazoxanide, azithromycin, chloroquine, ritonavir/lopinavir, and remdesivir can prevent viral entry, TMPRSS2, viral membrane fusion, endocytosis, and the RNA-dependent RNA polymerase. Monoclonal antibodies, PAC-MAN (widely known as prophylactic antiviral CRISPR in human cells), and designed recombinant soluble ACE2 are also considered additional therapies for VOCs.

Genomic monitoring/surveillance of SARS-CoV-2 variations is an additional strategy that will be used in the future to predict the pandemic at an early stage and initiate operative strategies to stop the propagation of SARS-CoV-2 variants and prevent the spread of other dangerous viruses. The effectiveness of current vaccinations varies, with some demonstrating diminished efficiency against VOCs. For protection against any virus or strain that belongs to a certain viral group, a universal vaccination is required. However, manufacturing such a vaccination requires new technologies and more investments. Identifying novel SARS-CoV-2 variants is critical for tracking the epidemic and viral progression. Current diagnostic assays identify specific viral genes or protein targets; however, mutations can reduce test sensitivity. Bacillus Calmette-Guerin (BCG) vaccination of children has been demonstrated to reduce COVID-19 cases and mortality rates globally. The BCG vaccine has been proven to enhance the immune system's ability to combat other bacteria, including tuberculosis.

Since the COVID-19 epidemic is the worst in a century, nations must cooperate to contain it. It is imperative that vaccines are distributed quickly, fairly, and with strong international coordination, all under the direction of the WHO. To avoid human contact and reverse zoonoses, animal immunizations are also required. It is vital to keep track of the progression of the illness and put in place a long-lasting strategy for the global genomic analysis of SARS-CoV-2. Because of the possibility of novel variations originating through interactions between the wild-type and vaccine strains, live attenuated vaccinations should be avoided.

Genomic monitoring is essential for assessing new variations and experimental statistics to calculate potential dangers. International procedures and legal frameworks are required for quick accessibility to viral components. The development of multivalent vaccinations against present and potential variations, the targeting of protein sequences with low mutation risk, and the pursuit of an ideal vaccine that is effective against all variant types, free of cold-chain restrictions, and noninjectable are some prospective possibilities.

10. Conclusions

A significant accomplishment is the development of effective vaccines against SARS-CoV-2 during the 16 months of the COVID-19 pandemic, with 95% effectiveness and 8.090 billion doses distributed across 184 countries. However, the emergence of variants, which is an indication of alarm, poses a serious challenge to tracking the pandemic's progress. The Omicron variant of SARS-CoV-2, along with five other significant mutations, have made it difficult to eradicate the virus. Recovery from the pandemic will take time because it has already had significant negative effects on the economy and public health. High-throughput technology and innovative vaccines will be required to address these problems, including multivalent vaccinations that provide long-term protection from all variants.

Abbreviations

ACE2	Angiotensin-converting enzyme 2
BCG	Bacillus Calmette-Guerin
DMVs	Double-membrane vesicles
ER	Endoplasmic Reticulum
ERGIC	Endoplasmic Reticulum-Golgi Intermediate Compartment
EUA	Emergency Use Authorization
GISAID	Global Initiative on Sharing All Influenza Data
gRNA	Genomic RNA
Mpro	Main Protease Inhibitor
NPIs	Nonpharmaceutical Interventions
NSP	Non-structural Protein
NTDs	Neglected Tropical Diseases
Plpro	Papain-like Protease
pp1a, pp1ab	Large Polyproteins
RBD	Receptor Binding Domain
RNA	Ribonucleic Acid
SA	South Africa
sgRNA	Sub-genomic RNA
TMPRSS2	Transmembrane Protease, Serine2
UK	United Kingdom
US	United States
USA	United States of America
VOC	Variants of Concern
VOI	Variants of Interest
WHO	World Health Organization

DOI: http://dx.doi.org/10.5772/intechopen.1003717

Author details

Ishrat Perveen[1*], Bakhtawar Bukhari[1], Naaz Abbas[1], Sania Mazhar[1], Yasar Saleem[1], Shaista Nawaz[1], Samia Nawab[2*], Quratulain Syed[1], Syed Hussain Imam Abidi[3], Sana Riaz[1], Ramsha Essa[1], Abad Ali Nadeem[1], Muhammad Farooq[1], Fatima Akram[1] and Saba Sabahat[4]

1 Food and Biotechnology Research Centre, Pakistan Council of Scientific and Industrial Research Centre, Lahore, Pakistan

2 Government Graduate College For Women, Township, Lahore, Pakistan

3 Pakistan Council of Scientific and Industrial Research Centre (PCSIR), Islamabad, Pakistan

4 Rashid Latif College of Pharmacy (RLCP), Lahore, Pakistan

*Address all correspondence to: drishratperveen51214@outlook.com, drishratperveen@outlook.com, drishratperveen51214@gmail.com and samianawab74@gmail.com

References

[1] Pagani I, Ghezzi S, Alberti S, Poli G, Vicenzi E. Origin and evolution of SARS-CoV-2. The European Physical Journal Plus. 2023;**138**:157. DOI: 10.1140/epjp/s13360-023-03719-6

[2] Li J, Jia H, Tian M, Wu N, Yang X, Qi J, et al. SARS-CoV-2 and emerging variants: Unmasking structure, function, infection, and immune escape mechanisms. Frontiers in Cellular and Infection Microbiology. 2022;**12**:3-4. DOI: 10.3389/fcimb.2022.869832

[3] Tabata K, Prasad V, Paul D, Lee J-Y, Pham M-T, Twu W-I, et al. Convergent use of phosphatidic acid for hepatitis C virus and SARS-CoV-2 replication organelle formation. Nature Communications. 2021;**12**:7276. DOI: 10.1038/s41467-021-27511-1

[4] Zhang H, Zhang H. Entry, egress and vertical transmission of SARS-CoV-2. Journal of Molecular Cell Biology. 2021;**13**:168-174. DOI: 10.1093/jmcb/mjab013

[5] Tegally H, Wilkinson E, Giovanetti M, Iranzadeh A, Fonseca V, Giandhari J, et al. Detection of a SARS-CoV-2 variant of concern in South Africa. Nature. 2021;**592**:438-443. DOI: 10.1038/s41586-021-03402-9

[6] Cascella M, Rajnik M, Aleem A, Dulebohn SC, Di Napoli R. Features, Evaluation, and Treatment of Coronavirus (COVID-19). 2023 Aug 18. In: StatPearls [Internet]. Treasure Island (FL): StatPearls Publishing; 2023 Jan–. PMID: 32150360

[7] Scovino AM, Dahab EC, Vieira GF, Freire-de-Lima L, Freire-de-Lima CG, Morrot A. SARS-CoV-2's variants of concern: A brief characterization. Frontiers in Immunology. 2022;**13**:6-7. DOI: 10.3389/fimmu.2022.834098

[8] Jeong GU, Yoon GY, Moon HW, Lee W, Hwang I, Kim H, et al. Comparison of plaque size, thermal stability, and replication rate among SARS-CoV-2 variants of concern. Viruses. 2021;**14**:55. DOI: 10.3390/v14010055

[9] Raja RK, Nguyen-Tri P, Balasubramani G, Alagarsamy A, Hazir S, Ladhari S, et al. SARS-CoV-2 and its new variants: A comprehensive review on nanotechnological application insights into potential approaches. Applied Nanoscience. 2023;**13**:65-93. DOI: 10.1007/s13204-021-01900-w

[10] Luban J, Sattler RA, Mühlberger E, Graci JD, Cao L, Weetall M, et al. The DHODH inhibitor PTC299 arrests SARS-CoV-2 replication and suppresses induction of inflammatory cytokines. Virus Research. 2021;**292**:198246. DOI: 10.1016/j.virusres.2020.198246

[11] Corti D, Purcell LA, Snell G, Veesler D. Tackling COVID-19 with neutralizing monoclonal antibodies. Cell. 2021;**184**:3086-3108. DOI: 10.1016/j.cell.2021.05.005

[12] Şimşek Yavuz S, Komşuoğlu Çelikyurt İ. An update of anti-viral treatment of COVID-19. Turk. Journal of Medical Sciences. 2021;**51**:3372-3390. DOI: 10.3906/sag-2106-250

[13] Caly L, Druce JD, Catton MG, Jans DA, Wagstaff KM. The FDA-approved drug ivermectin inhibits the replication of SARS-CoV-2 in vitro. Antiviral Research. 2020;**178**:104787. DOI: 10.1016/j.antiviral.2020.104787

[14] Alavi Darazam I, Shokouhi S, Pourhoseingholi MA, Naghibi Irvani SS,

Mokhtari M, Shabani M, et al. Role of interferon therapy in severe COVID-19: The COVIFERON randomized controlled trial. Scientific Reports. 2021;**11**:8059. DOI: 10.1038/s41598-021-86859-y

[15] London School of Hygiene & Tropical Medicine. COVID-19 Vaccine Tracker. https://Vac-LshtmShinyappsIo/Ncov_vaccine_landscape/

[16] Ling Y, Zhong J, Luo J. Safety and effectiveness of SARS-CoV-2 vaccines: A systematic review and meta-analysis. Journal of Medical Virology. 2021;**93**:6486-6495. DOI: 10.1002/jmv.27203

[17] Zhang J, Zeng H, Gu J, Li H, Zheng L, Zou Q. Progress and prospects on vaccine development against SARS-CoV-2. Vaccines (Basel). 2020;**8**:153. DOI: 10.3390/vaccines8020153

[18] Backer V, Sjöbring U, Sonne J, Weiss A, Hostrup M, Johansen HK, et al. A randomized, double-blind, placebo-controlled phase 1 trial of inhaled and intranasal niclosamide: A broad spectrum antiviral candidate for treatment of COVID-19. The Lancet Regional Health - Europe. 2021;**4**:100084. DOI: 10.1016/j.lanepe.2021.100084

Chapter 4

Understanding the Omicron Variant in the COVID-19 Pandemic

Safae El Mazouri, Tarik Aanniz, Sara Louati, Lahcen Belyamani, Rachid El Jaoudi and Mouna Ouadghiri

Abstract

The proposed chapter aims to provide an overview of the severe acute respiratory syndrome coronavirus 2 (SARS-CoV-2) Omicron variant and its potential effects on public health. The origins of coronavirus disease of 2019 (COVID-19) pandemic and the SARS-CoV-2 virus evolution through time will be briefly covered at the beginning of the chapter with an emphasis on the emergence of new variants. The next section will present an overview of Omicron, outlining where it was first identified, the key mutations that set it apart from prior variants, and how it has spread worldwide. In the following section, we will briefly discuss the evidence regarding Omicron's rapid spread in comparison to other COVID-19 variants along with any possible implications in disease severity and hospitalization rates. The chapter also explores how Omicron could affect natural immunity and vaccination efficiency and will provide information on recent studies on the effectiveness of COVID-19 vaccines against Omicron. Finally, we will discuss public health responses to Omicron's emergence and outline the effective strategies that can lessen its effects.

Keywords: SARS-CoV-2, Omicron, variant of concern, COVID-19, pandemic

1. Introduction

The COVID-19 pandemic, caused by the SARS-CoV-2 virus, is believed to have originated in a seafood market in the city of Wuhan, China, in late 2019. The World Health Organization (WHO) declared the COVID-19 outbreak a global pandemic on March 11, 2020. The exact origin and transmission route of the virus are still under investigation by the scientific community, but it is believed to have originated in bats and may have been transmitted to humans through an intermediate host, possibly a pangolin [1, 2].

The SARS-CoV-2 virus has quickly spread to other parts of China and then to other countries around the world. The rapid and wide expansion of the virus was facilitated by its ability to be transmitted through respiratory droplets [3], and by the fact that infected individuals can exhibit mild symptoms or be entirely asymptomatic, thereby complicating efforts to identify and control its spread [4].

As of May 2023, the virus has infected more than 700 million people and caused almost 7 million deaths worldwide [5]. The pandemic has had a profound impact on the world, resulting in substantial disruptions across social and economic domains. Moreover, it has underscored the critical significance of preparedness in addressing future outbreaks of infectious diseases [6].

Like all viruses, SARS-CoV-2 can mutate as it replicates. Mutations are changes in the virus's genetic material (RNA) that occur randomly and can result in new variants with different characteristics. Most of these mutations are harmless, but some may make the virus more infectious or resistant to immune responses [7].

Since the beginning of the pandemic, numerous SARS-CoV-2 variants have emerged, including the Alpha, Beta, Gamma, Delta, and Omicron variants [8]. These variants differ from the original strain of the virus in key genetic changes that affect the virus's Spike (S) protein, which is used by the virus to infect human cells [9].

The Omicron variant was first identified in South Africa in November 2021. It has more than 50 mutations in its S protein, including many in the receptor-binding domain (RBD), which is the part of the S protein that attaches to human cells. Some of these mutations are similar to those seen in other variants, such as Delta, but others are unique to Omicron [10, 11].

These mutations are believed to make the virus more infectious and may also help it evade the immune system, including antibodies generated by vaccination or a previous infection [12]. According to preliminary findings, the Omicron variant has a greater risk of re-infection than the other variants. In South Africa, hospitalization rates are increased, and fewer people who needed oxygen support were presenting less severe symptoms as compared to previous variants [13].

It is important to note that SARS-CoV-2 will continue to evolve and mutate over time, and new variants may continue to emerge. Therefore, ongoing surveillance and research are critical to understand the impact of these variants and to develop effective strategies in order to control the spread of the virus and protect public health [14].

2. Overview of Omicron

Omicron (B.1.1.529) was first identified in Botswana, South Africa, and was classified on November 26, 2021, as a "variant of concern" by the World Health Organization due to its high number of mutations and potential impact on public health [10].

It was reported that Omicron was spreading at a much faster rate than Delta variant, with a basic reproduction number (R0) estimated to be 8.2. This means that each infected person could potentially transmit the virus to eight people [15].

The emergence of the Omicron variant has caused a new wave of infections with high hospitalization rates worldwide. This wave is distinct from those caused by earlier variants, and its peak is significantly higher [16]. Apart from B.1.1.529, multiple sub-lineages have been identified and studied, with over 100 subvariants estimated to exist. Among these subvariants are BA.1 and its sister-variant BA.2, and other diverse Omicron variants, such as BA.4, BA.5, BA.2.12.1, BA.2.75, BA.2.75.2, BQ.1, BQ.1.1, and BF.7. Additionally, several recombinant subvariants of Omicron, including XBB, XBB.1.5, and XBB.1.16, have emerged [17]. These subvariants exhibit unique characteristics and have been linked to diverse epidemiological patterns [18].

Sequencing analysis revealed that Omicron variant harbors several key mutations that differentiate it from earlier variants like Delta. BA.1 is a variant of concern due to its high number of mutations in the S gene, particularly in the receptor-binding domain and the N-terminal domain. These mutations can impact ACE2 binding and antibody recognition. The variant shares the deletion at positions S:H69- and S:V70- with Alpha and Eta, among others. It is noteworthy that del69-70 in the S protein is being explored as a diagnostic marker for Omicron, as the TaqPath PCR test yields negative results for the S gene in this variant but positive results for other SARS-CoV-2 variants [19]. There is a 3 amino-acid insertion ('EPE') at position 214 in the S protein, which is located in an area known as an "insertion hotspot" [20–23]. A cluster of mutations at the S1-S2 furin cleavage site (S:H655Y, S:N679K, S:P681H) may be associated with increased transmissibility. The mutation at S:E484A is also present in other variants and mutations at this position have been linked to immune escape. The combination of mutations S:Q498R and S:N501Y has been shown to significantly enhance the binding affinity to ACE2 in *in-vitro* evolution studies [24, 25]. Additionally, there is a three amino-acid deletion in ORF1a at ORF1a:L3674-, ORF1a:S3675-, and ORF1a:G3676-. This deletion may affect innate immune evasion by compromising cells' ability to degrade viral components [26]. The accessory protein ORF9b has a three amino-acid deletion at ORF9b:E27-, ORF9b:N28-, and ORF9b:A29-. ORF9b is believed to suppress the innate immune response by interacting with TOM70 and NEMO, ultimately impacting interferon production [27–29]. Lastly, two ancestral mutations in the Nucleocapsid protein, N:R203K and N:G204R, have been associated with increased subgenomic RNA expression and higher viral loads [30, 31]. Moreover, BA.2 and BA.1 share 38 mutations in both nucleotides and amino acids. However, BA.2 has an additional 27 unique mutations, while BA.1 has an additional 20 unique mutations. In the S protein alone, both variants share 21 amino acid mutations. BA.1 has 12 additional unique amino acid mutations, while BA.2 has six additional unique amino acid mutations, along with a deletion/mutation. It is important to note that BA.2 lacks the deletion del69-70. The six additional Spike mutations in BA.2 are S:T19I, S:V213G, S:S371F, S:T376A, S:D405N, and S:R408S. Additionally, there is a nine-nucleotide deletion (position 21,633–21,641) that leads to the deletions and mutation S:L24-, S:P25-, S:P26-, and S:A27S. The ORF1a:L3201F mutation has emerged multiple times within BA.2. In South Africa, where the variant is suspected to have originated, it is mostly present in its wild-type form. However, outside of South Africa, the ORF1a:L3201F mutation is more common. Therefore, sub-clades of BA.2 may or may not have the ORF1a:L3201F mutation depending on their lineage. The variant BA.4 appears to have arisen in late 2021, while BA.5 likely arose in early 2022. Both variant sequences were predominantly from South Africa, though now are detected globally. BA.4 and BA.5 have identical Spike proteins, leading researchers to group them together in studies focusing on Spike alone, such as antibody research. These variants share several Spike mutations with BA.1 and even more Spike mutations with BA.2. In fact, the Spike mutations in BA.2, BA.4, and BA.5 are mostly identical. The only difference is that BA.4 and BA.5 lack the S:Q493R mutation found in BA.2 and instead have S:L452R and S:F486V mutations. Furthermore, they share the deletion del69-70 with BA.1, which allows BA.4 and BA.5 to be detected through "S gene drop out" or "S gene target failure (SGTF)" in certain qPCR assays [32]. It is noteworthy that BA.4 and BA.5 formed >50% of the subvariants during June–July 2022 [33].

The BA.2.12.1 variant shares many Spike mutations with both BA.1 and BA.2 variants. Specifically, the Spike mutations of BA.2 and BA.2.12.1 are identical, except that BA.2.12.1 has two additional mutations at S:L452Q and S:S704L. In terms of amino-acid mutations outside of Spike, BA.2.12.1 does not have any additional mutations compared to BA.2. In South Africa, where this variant is believed to have originated, the wild type is most prevalent. Outside of South Africa, the ORF1a:L3201F mutation is more common. Therefore, sub-clades of BA.2 may or may not have the ORF1a:L3201F mutation, depending on whether they are descended from a part of BA.2 carrying this mutation. It is worth noting that the BA.4 and BA.5 variants, thought to have emerged in South Africa, do not possess this mutation, whereas BA.2.12.1, believed to have originated in North America, does have it. It is noteworthy that neutralizing titers against BA.2.12.1 were lower in vaccinated individuals who received the CoronaVac vaccine compared to BA.2. Additionally, BA.2.12.1 showed an increased affinity for binding to ACE2 receptors compared to BA.1 and other variants [34].

The variant BA.2.75 seems to have emerged in late spring 2022, potentially originating in India. By July 2022, most of the identified sequences of this lineage were found in India, but it has also been detected in various countries globally. BA.2.75 shares many Spike mutations with BA.1 and BA.2. It has the same Spike mutations as its parent, BA.2, except for S:G446S and S:R493Q, and it has additional mutations: S:K147E, S:W152R, S:F157L, S:I210V, S:G257S, S:G339H, and S:N460K. It does not have the MutationS:H69- and S:V70-deletion found in BA.4 and BA.2.12.1. Adintrevimab, bamlanivimab, casirivimab, and etesevimab were not effective against BA.2.75, but ragdanvimab, sotrovimab, and tixagevimab were effective. However, BA.2.75 showed higher resistance against cilgavimab and bebtelovimab compared to BA.2 [35]. BA.2.75 is more immune-evasive than BA.4/BA.5 in areas with previous Delta infection and may escape BA.2-induced immunity. It may also have higher ACE-2 binding affinity than BA.4/ BA.5 [36]. A study using donated blood from Sweden did not find greater immune evasion by BA.2.75 compared to BA.5 [37]. BA.2.75 subvariant was undergoing further mutations and forming a new subvariant known as BA.2.75.2, it comprises specific substitutions such as R346T, F486S, and D1199N, along with S:K444T and S:N460K [38].

BQ.1 variant probably emerged in mid-2022, potentially in central or western Africa. It gained attention in August as a notable variant and has since spread worldwide. BQ.1 shares all the mutations found in BA.5 but also has additional mutations. Within Spike, it has mutations at S:K444T and S:N460K, and the S:Q493R mutation found in its ancestor, BA.2, is reverted to S:Q493Q in BQ.1. Outside of Spike, it has mutations at ORF1a:Q556K, ORF1a:L3829F, ORF1b:Y264H, ORF1b:M1156I, ORF9b:P10F, and N:E136D. There is concern that BQ.1 may have an increased ability to evade existing immunity. Studies have shown a significant reduction in neutralization titers against BQ.1, especially in sublineage BQ.1.1, indicating the potential for immune escape. It can also escape certain monoclonal antibodies, making them likely ineffective against the variant. The mutation S:N460K is associated with neutralizing antibody evasion and is driving enhanced neutralization resistance and fusogenicity in BQ.1 and BQ.1.1 lineages [39–41]. Since late September 2022, China has been experiencing a continuous increase in COVID-19 cases, and this resurgence can be attributed to the emergence of a subvariant known as SARS-CoV-2 Omicron BF.7 (BA.5.2.1.7), which is a subtype of BA.5. This particular subvariant has been detected in several countries, including Belgium, China, Denmark, Norway, France, Germany, India, Mongolia, the United Kingdom (UK), and the United States (US) [42, 43]. The heightened transmission rate of the BF.7 subvariant can be attributed to the presence of novel mutations in its spike protein. Molecular modeling studies have shed light on how these mutations, namely K444T, F486S, and D1199N, affect the RBD of the spike protein, enabling antibody-mediated immune evasion. Additionally, BF.7 carries an additional mutation, R346T, in the spike protein, which is derived from the BA.4/5 subvariant. This specific mutation contributes to a 4.4-fold increase in resistance to neutralization compared to the original D614G variant. Notably, the R346T mutation in the BF.7 variant's spike glycoprotein, especially within the RBD, has been associated with a heightened ability to evade neutralizing antibodies generated by vaccines or previous infections [43].

XBB is a recombinant variant composed of genetic material from two different parent variants, lineage BJ.1 and BM.1.1.1, parts of BA.2 and BA.2.75, respectively, with a breakpoint in the S1 region of the Spike subunit. The initial sequences were identified in August 2022 and originated from India. Since then, it has experienced significant global expansion. It has unique mutations S:V445P from BJ.1 and S:N460K from BM.1.1.1. This recombination likely occurred within a short region containing these mutations. Before the breakpoint, XBB carries all the mutations of its BJ.1 parent, and after the breakpoint, it carries all the mutations of its BM.1.1.1 parent. It also shares common mutations with the broader BA.2 lineage. Additional mutations found in XBB include S:V83A, S:Y144-, S:H146Q, S:Q183E, S:V213E, S:G339H, S:R346T, S:L386I, S:G446S, S:F486S, and S:F490S. It also has a unique synonymous mutation at A19326G.

Certain sublineages within XBB, such as XBB.1, have acquired additional amino acid mutations S:G252V and ORF8:G8*, which raise concerns about its ability to evade existing immunity.

Preliminary laboratory results indicate that XBB may have a higher potential to evade immune responses. A study showed a significant reduction in neutralization titers against XBB in vaccinated individuals while maintaining ACE2 binding affinity. It was also found that clinically available monoclonal antibodies Evusheld and Bebtelovimab are likely ineffective against XBB, and sublineage XBB.1 escaped all NTD-targeting neutralizing antibodies tested [39].

XBB.1.5 is a recombinant variant that descends from XBB, likely arose by October 2022, possibly in North America. As a result, XBB.1.5 shares the same mutations as XBB, along with a few additional mutations, including S:G252V and ORF8:G8*. Additionally, XBB.1.5 has a nucleotide mutation at position T23018C, which causes the S:F486S mutation in XBB to change to S:F486P. This change from S to P in the Spike protein has implications for ACE2 binding. Based on the Spike protein mutations in XBB.1.5, it is expected to have similar immune evasion properties as its parental lineages, XBB.1 and XBB, but with the potential for enhanced transmission due to the new S:F486P mutation. Studies have shown that neutralizing titers in vaccinated individuals with breakthrough infections were comparable between XBB.1 and XBB.1.5, but ACE2 binding was significantly stronger in XBB.1.5, suggesting a potential growth advantage for XBB.1.5 over XBB and XBB.1 [44]. Another study found minimal differences in neutralizing titers and fusogenicity among XBB, XBB.1, and 23A XBB.1.5 in vaccinated/infected individuals [45]. Furthermore, neutralizing antibody titers were similar between XBB.1.5 and XBB.1 in a study involving bivalently-boosted mRNA vaccine recipients [46].

The variant XBB.1.16 is descended from variant XBB. It likely emerged towards the end of 2022 or the beginning of 2023, possibly in Asia. XBB.1.16 shares the same mutations as XBB, with additional mutations including S:G252V and ORF8:G8*, as well as ORF1a:L3829F, ORF1b:D1746Y, ORF9b:I5T, and ORF9b:N55S.

Similar to XBB.1.5, XBB.1.16 has an additional nucleotide mutation resulting in the S:F486S mutation in XBB becoming S:F486P. This change affects ACE2 binding. Additionally, XBB.1.16 has unique synonymous mutations at T12730A, A14856G, and C29386T.

Based on the Spike protein mutations, XBB.1.16 is expected to have immune evasion properties similar to its parental lineages, XBB.1 and XBB, potentially enhanced by the S:F486P mutation and the RBD mutation S:T478R. The impact of the Spike mutation S:E180V is less certain.

Preliminary studies suggest that XBB.1.16 may evade immunity, similar to XBB.1.5, based on neutralizing titers against mRNA-vaccinated individuals with breakthrough BA.2/BA.5 infections. XBB.1.16 shows resistance to most monoclonal antibodies, except strovimab [47]. Binding affinity to the ACE2 receptor may be lower than XBB.1.5 but higher than XBB.1. It is estimated to have a higher reproductive number compared to XBB.1.5 and XBB.1 [47]. Early reports from India have indicated changing demographic and clinical associations with XBB.1.16 infections, including cases of conjunctivitis [48]. The WHO designated XBB.1.16 as a Variant of Interest (VOI) on April 17, 2023 [49].

3. Clinical characteristics and severity

The burden of COVID-19 on hospital services is determined by the prevalence and severity of SARS-CoV-2 variants, and modified by individual factors such as age, frailty, and vaccination status [50, 51].

Despite Omicron displaying only mild severity, its 3.31 times greater transmission rate than the Delta variant represents a global epidemic threat [52]. The clinical presentation of the Omicron variant differs from previous SARS-CoV-2 variants. The most common symptoms are a cough, runny nose, congestion, and fatigue. A sore throat and a hoarse voice were more prevalent during the Omicron outbreak. Individuals infected with Omicron are less likely to show at least one of the three classic symptoms of COVID-19: the loss of smell, a fever, and a persistent cough, which are associated with individuals infected with the Delta variant [53]. The Omicron variant outbreak has also resulted in a large number of asymptomatic carriers, which may have resulted in milder symptoms. In all age groups, respiratory discomfort is a typical sign. Vomiting is the most typical gastroenterological symptom, and children with Omicron infection aged 5–9 years old also frequently experience diarrhea and abdominal pains [54]. Children in the age group of 9–11 show less severe symptoms than infants do, which is valid for both Delta and Omicron variants [55]. The Omicron variant exhibited a lower replication rate in lung and gut cell lines but replicated faster in primary cultures of human nasal epithelial cells. Omicron has been reported to multiply faster in human airway organoids and *ex vivo* bronchus explant cultures, but less efficiently in human alveoli organoids and *ex vivo* lung explant cultures [56, 57]. These findings indicated that Omicron infected the upper respiratory system rather than the lungs, which might result in enhanced transmissibility and a better prognosis.

Across multiple studies, it has been consistently observed that Omicron-infected patients have lower hospital admission rates compared to other variants, regardless of their vaccination status or number of vaccine doses. Specifically, lower ICU admission rates have been reported among Omicron-infected patients compared to other variants, irrespective of vaccination status or vaccine doses. Moreover, Omicron-infected patients exhibit lower rates of oxygen therapies [58].

Empirical evidence from real-world scenarios indicates that vaccine effectiveness against symptomatic disease caused by the Omicron variant is lower and tends to deteriorate faster over time than with the Delta variant [59, 60]. However, Omicron infection still resulted in substantial patient and public health burden and an increased hospital admission rate of older patients with Omicron, which counteracts some of the benefit arising from less severe disease [61–65].

4. Immunity and vaccination

Vaccine effectiveness against severe diseases is a matter of concern. The vaccine's effectiveness is not largely affected by the variants. This is because of the mutations of the variants, which hinder the neutralization potency of any vaccine. In the Omicron case, several mutations have been noted in the nAb binding region of the S protein, especially in RBD and NTD, which cause the nAb escape phenomenon. Therefore, we can say that the Omicron variant possesses a partial vaccine escape ability [23, 66].

Recent studies elucidate that the Omicron sub-lineages, BA.1, BA.2, and BA.3, are very competent in escaping the immune system. The subjects who have taken one or two doses of the vaccine cannot protect against these variants significantly, thus, the neutralization efficiency of the vaccines is gradually decreasing. Most surprisingly, people who had received three shots of the vaccine only have partial protection from the infection of these variants [41, 67, 68]. Moreover, certain Omicron subvariants such as BA.4.6, BF.7, BQ.1, BQ.1.1, and BA.2.75.2 displayed some level of enhanced neutralization resistance compared to their parental subvariants. Among them, BQ.1, BQ.1.1, and BA.2.75.2 demonstrated the strongest resistance [69]. These findings are consistent with another research where the sensitivity of BA.2.75.2, BA.4.6, and BQ.1.1 to six therapeutic monoclonal antibodies (mAbs) and 72 sera samples from individuals vaccinated with Pfizer BNT162b2 was investigated. It was observed that Ronapreve (Casirivimab and Imdevimab) and Evusheld (Cilgavimab and Tixagevimab) lost their antiviral effectiveness against BA.2.75.2 and BQ.1.1 subvariants, while Xevudy (Sotrovimab) exhibited limited activity. Additionally, BQ.1.1 showed resistance to Bebtelovimab. The neutralizing titers in individuals who received three vaccine doses were either low or undetectable against BQ.1.1 and BA.2.75.2, four months after the booster shot. However, a breakthrough infection with BA.1/BA.2 led to an increase in these titers, albeit remaining about 18-fold lower against BA.2.75.2 and BQ.1.1 compared to BA.1. Conversely, a breakthrough infection with BA.5 resulted in a more efficient increase in neutralization against BA.5 and BQ.1.1 than against BA.2.75.2 [38]. Importantly, it was observed that the neutralization resistance of BQ.1 and BQ.1.1 was primarily driven by the N460K mutation, while the resistance of the BA.2.75.2 subvariant was determined by the F486S mutation. The N460K mutation was identified to enhance ACE2 interactions, potentially leading to increased cell-cell fusion and neutralization resistance when introduced into BA.4/5-derived subvariants [69]. Furthermore, it has been shown that the mutations R346T, K444T, and F486S play a crucial role in antibody recognition and potentially contribute to immune evasion through these specific alterations. Significantly, these mutations not only conferred resistance to sera induced by 3-dose mRNA vaccines but also to sera from individuals previously infected with BA.1 and BA.4/5 variants [70].

Vaccine escape is a common phenomenon. Several researchers urge the development of new vaccines against the Omicron variant. The study conducted by Pérez-Then et al. evaluated the effect of a heterologous BNT162b2 mRNA vaccine booster on the humoral immunity of individuals who had previously received two doses of CoronaVac vaccine. The results showed that the heterologous CoronaVac prime followed by BNT162b2 booster induced high levels of virus-specific antibodies and potent neutralization activity against the SARS-CoV-2 Wuhan virus and Delta variant. However, neutralization activity against the Omicron variant was undetectable in those who had received two doses of CoronaVac. Following the BNT162b2 booster, neutralization activity against Omicron increased by 1.4-fold compared to two doses of mRNA vaccine, but the neutralizing antibody titers were still lower for Omicron compared to Wuhan virus and Delta variant. These findings suggest that countries using CoronaVac vaccines should consider mRNA vaccine boosters to combat the spread of Omicron and future emerging variants [71].

Rössler et al. conducted a study to evaluate the effectiveness of COVID-19 vaccines (mRNA-1273, ChAdOx1-S, and BNT162b2) against the Omicron variant. The results showed that individuals vaccinated with these vaccines had much lower neutralization levels against the Omicron variant compared to other variants (Alpha, Beta, or Delta). However, cross-neutralization persisted in individuals who had received the BNT162b2 vaccine or a heterologous ChAdOx1-S-BNT162b2 vaccine but not in those who had received the homologous ChAdOx1-S vaccine. Serum samples obtained from individuals who had received the mRNA-1273 vaccine 4–6 months after the second dose did not show any neutralizing antibodies against the omicron variant, but the interval between the second dose and sample collection was longer than for other vaccination-regimen groups [72].

A test-negative case-control study found that receiving three doses of mRNA COVID-19 vaccine was associated with protection against symptomatic infection caused by the SARS-CoV-2 Omicron and Delta variants. The study analyzed 70,155 tests from symptomatic adults and concluded that a third dose of the mRNA vaccine can increase the vaccine's protective efficacy against both variants [73].

Lee and colleagues showed that previous infection in octogenarians followed by two doses of BNT162b2 resulted in strong neutralization of the omicron variant when compared to subjects who had only received two BNT162b2 doses [74]. In addition, a separate study measured the neutralization potency of serum from individuals who received two doses of mRNA-1273 or BNT162b2 vaccines or one dose of Ad26.COV2.S vaccine against Wuhan virus, Delta, and Omicron pseudoviruses [75].

Currently, several researchers or pharmacological companies have developed new vaccines against the Omicron variant [76]. ModernaTX has developed two mRNA-based bivalent vaccines, notably mRNA-1273.214 [77] and mRNA-1273.222. The safety and efficacy of the vaccine have been evaluated through a total of seven clinical trials and was approved in 38 and 33 countries, respectively. In addition to ModernaTX's bivalent vaccine, Pfizer-BioNTech has also created a bivalent COVID-19 vaccine. Pfizer-BioNTech has developed the BNT162b2 (B.1.1.529) and BNT162b2 Bivalent (covid19.trackvaccines.org). A total of seven clinical trials have been conducted to understand these vaccines' safety profile, ultimately, they were approved in more than 35 and 33 countries, respectively. These two bivalent vaccines' safety profiles have also been assessed in kidney transplant recipients [78].

These findings highlight the worrisome evolutionary path of the Omicron subvariants, enabling their transmission in vaccinated populations, and raise concerns about the efficacy of most available monoclonal antibodies.

5. Public health responses

The continuous emergence of new variants of SARS-CoV-2 has consistently raised significant global public health concerns, leading to waves of the COVID-19 pandemic. This ongoing crisis has obliged countries to establish and maintain comprehensive public health measures aimed at detecting and managing emerging infectious threats. The unprecedented magnitude and duration of the pandemic have appropriately sparked inquiries into the key elements necessary for a strong and sustainable public health response [79]. The extent of the threat posed by the Omicron variant is primarily determined by four crucial inquiries: (i) the level of transmissibility exhibited by the variant, (ii) the effectiveness of vaccines and previous infection in preventing a new infection, transmission, clinical illness, and mortality, (iii) the virulence of the variant in comparison to other variants, and (iv) the population's comprehension of these dynamics, their perception of risk, and adherence to control measures, including public health and social measures [80].

In order to mitigate the transmission of Omicron and other emerging variants, it is crucial to implement proposed preventive measures diligently, taking into account the lessons learned from previous waves of the COVID-19 pandemic. This includes conducting widespread confirmatory diagnosis, as well as global genomic surveillance and sequencing of a larger number of SARS-CoV-2 isolates. In-depth studies are needed to understand the higher transmissibility and pathogenicity acquired by emerging variants, focusing on SARS-CoV-2-host interactions, adaptation, evolutionary dynamics, and mechanisms of genomic mutation or variation. Strengthening medical research facilities and trained staff for gene sequencing, variant identification, and characterization is essential, along with a collaborative global approach to update genomic and epidemiological data repositories. These efforts will contribute to a more effective response to emerging variants [11, 81–85].

To safeguard the health of the global population and achieve herd immunity, it is important to enhance COVID-19 vaccination drives with equitable global access, wider acceptance, and reduced vaccine hesitancy. However, long-term protection and the attainment of herd immunity still face threats from the adverse effects of emerging variants on vaccine efficacy and protective immunity. The evaluation and adequate addressing of these challenges are necessary. COVID-19 vaccines, such as BNT162b2, mRNA-1273, CoronaVac, Sputnik V, and AZD1222, have demonstrated varying levels of prevention and protection against severe COVID-19 caused by VOCs. Strategic planning should prioritize the strengthening of vaccination efforts with highly effective vaccines and booster doses to limit the virus's ability to acquire mutations. This is particularly important in low-income countries, where slow or delayed vaccination approaches could leave a larger susceptible population [86–88].

Strict adherence to recommended public health measures, including COVID-19-appropriate behaviors such as social distancing, wearing face masks, practicing hand hygiene, restricting movements, and avoiding mass gatherings, is crucial in preventing SARS-CoV-2 infection and the spread of variants. Special attention should be given to vulnerable groups, including the unvaccinated, elderly individuals, and those with underlying illnesses, to minimize the risk of infection and disease transmission. Making vaccination compulsory and emphasizing the importance of vaccination/immunization certificates for travel and crossing international borders can act as a protective measure against community transmission of emerging variants and mutants of SARS-CoV-2. Evaluating the transmissibility, severity, diagnostic test sensitivity and specificity, vaccine efficacy, and treatment effectiveness will aid in effectively addressing Omicron and future variant outbreaks [89, 90].

In response to the Omicron variant, many countries have implemented travel restrictions and other measures to limit the importation of new cases. The WHO and other health organizations are closely monitoring the situation and have established a global surveillance network to track the spread of the variant and coordinate efforts to contain the virus. Ongoing research is being conducted to understand the characteristics of the Omicron variant and develop new strategies to prevent and treat COVID-19, including new vaccines and treatments specifically designed for the variant. To support these efforts, the WHO has established a global task force to ensure equitable distribution of vaccines and treatments to all countries, particularly those with limited resources. Overall, the response to the Omicron variant has been a coordinated global effort to protect public health [91].

6. Conclusion

In conclusion, the emergence of the Omicron variant in the ongoing COVID-19 pandemic has presented us with new challenges and uncertainties. Throughout this chapter, we have explored the key aspects of Omicron, including its overview, severity, transmissibility, vaccination, immunity, and public health responses.

Omicron has demonstrated a higher degree of transmissibility compared to previous variants, leading to rapid surges in infection rates across the globe. The concerns surrounding the Omicron variant stem from its potential to evade specific immune responses and potentially diminish the efficacy of current vaccines. Nevertheless, it is important to emphasize the necessity of ongoing research and analysis in order to comprehensively grasp the implications of this variant.

The development and administration of effective vaccines remain crucial tools in our fight against COVID-19, including the Omicron variant. Vaccination efforts should be prioritized, focusing on optimizing booster doses and adapting existing vaccines to enhance their efficacy against emerging variants. Continued research and development will be essential in this pursuit, ensuring our ability to adapt and counter future challenges.

Public health responses have played a pivotal role in mitigating the impact of the pandemic, and this remains true for Omicron. Enhanced surveillance, testing, and contact tracing efforts are essential for early detection and containment. Swift and evidence-based policy decisions, including targeted restrictions and public health messaging, can help prevent further spread and protect vulnerable populations.

Despite the challenges posed by the Omicron variant, it is important to maintain a balanced perspective. Scientific advancements, global collaboration, and lessons learned from previous waves of the pandemic have equipped us with valuable tools and knowledge. By applying these insights, we can navigate this new phase of the pandemic with resilience and resolve.

In conclusion, our understanding of the Omicron variant is still evolving. Vigilance, flexibility, and a commitment to evidence-based decision-making will be crucial in managing its impact.

Acknowledgements

The author would like to acknowledge the support received from the National Center for Scientific and Technical Research in Morocco through the Scholarship of Excellence.

Conflict of interest

The authors declare no conflict of interest.

Author details

Safae El Mazouri[1], Tarik Aanniz[1], Sara Louati[1], Lahcen Belyamani[2,3,4], Rachid El Jaoudi[1,2,5] and Mouna Ouadghiri[1*]

1 Medical Biotechnology Laboratory, Medical and Pharmacy School, Mohammed V University, Rabat, Morocco

2 Centre Mohammed VI of Research and Innovation (CM6), Rabat, Morocco

3 Mohammed VI University of Health Sciences (UM6SS), Casablanca, Morocco

4 Emergency Department, Military Hospital Mohammed V, Medical and Pharmacy School, Mohammed V University, Rabat, Morocco

5 Pharmacology and Toxicology Department, Medical and Pharmacy School, Mohammed V University, Rabat, Morocco

*Address all correspondence to: m.ouadghiri@um5r.ac.ma

References

[1] Hui DS, Azhar EI, Madani TA, et al. The continuing 2019-nCoV epidemic threat of novel coronaviruses to global health—The latest 2019 novel coronavirus outbreak in Wuhan, China. International Journal of Infectious Diseases. 2020;**91**:264-266. DOI: 10.1016/j.ijid.2020.01.009

[2] Saxena SK, Kumar S, Ansari S, et al. Transmission dynamics and mutational prevalence of the novel severe acute respiratory syndrome coronavirus-2 omicron variant of concern. Journal of Medical Virology. 2022;**94**(5):2160-2166. DOI: 10.1002/jmv.27611

[3] Lotfi M, Hamblin MR, Rezaei N. COVID-19: Transmission, prevention, and potential therapeutic opportunities. Clinica Chimica Acta. 2020;**508**:254-266. DOI: 10.1016/j.cca.2020.05.044

[4] Chen N, Zhou M, Dong X, et al. Epidemiological and clinical characteristics of 99 cases of 2019 novel coronavirus pneumonia in Wuhan, China: A descriptive study. Lancet. 2020;**395**(10223):507-513. DOI: 10.1016/S0140-6736(20)30211-7

[5] WHO Coronavirus (COVID-19) Dashboard | WHO Coronavirus (COVID-19) Dashboard With Vaccination Data. Available from: https://covid19.who.int/ [Accessed: June 11, 2023]

[6] Hiscott J, Alexandridi M, Muscolini M, et al. The global impact of the coronavirus pandemic. Cytokine & Growth Factor Reviews. 2020;**53**:1-9. DOI: 10.1016/j.cytogfr.2020.05.010

[7] Akkiz H. Implications of the novel mutations in the SARS-CoV-2 genome for transmission, disease severity, and the vaccine development. Frontiers in Medicine (Lausanne). 2021;**8**:636532. DOI: 10.3389/fmed.2021.636532

[8] El Mazouri S, Bendani H, Boumajdi N, et al. Phylogeography and genomic analysis of sars-cov-2 delta variant in Morocco. Journal of Infection in Developing Countries. 2022;**16**:1258-1268

[9] Tomaszewski T, DeVries RS, Dong M, et al. New pathways of mutational change in SARS-CoV-2 proteomes involve regions of intrinsic disorder important for virus replication and release. Evolutionary Bioinformatics Online. 2020;**16**:1176934320965149. DOI: 10.1177/1176934320965149

[10] El Mazouri S, Bendani H, Boumajdi N, et al. Report of SARS-CoV-2 BA.1 Lineage in Morocco. Microbiology Resource Announcements. 2022;**11**(5):e0016922. DOI: 10.1128/mra.00169-22

[11] Ahmad SU, Hafeez Kiani B, Abrar M, et al. A comprehensive genomic study, mutation screening, phylogenetic and statistical analysis of SARS-CoV-2 and its variant omicron among different countries. Journal of Infection and Public Health. 2022;**15**(8):878-891. DOI: 10.1016/j.jiph.2022.07.002

[12] Syed AM, Ciling A, Taha TY, et al. Omicron mutations enhance infectivity and reduce antibody neutralization of SARS-CoV-2 virus-like particles. Preprint. medRxiv. 2022. DOI: 10.1101/2021.12.20.21268048

[13] Ren S-Y, Wang W-B, Gao R-D, et al. Omicron variant (B.1.1.529) of SARS-CoV-2: Mutation, infectivity, transmission, and vaccine resistance. World Journal of Clinical Cases.

2022;**10**(1):1-11. DOI: 10.12998/wjcc.v10.i1.1

[14] Rochman ND, Wolf YI, Faure G, et al. Ongoing global and regional adaptive evolution of SARS-CoV-2. bioRxiv. 2021:2020.10.12.336644. DOI: 10.1101/2020.10.12.336644

[15] Liu Y, Rocklöv J. The effective reproductive number of the Omicron variant of SARS-CoV-2 is several times relative to Delta. Journal of Travel Medicine. 2022;**29**(3):taac037. DOI: 10.1093/jtm/taac037

[16] Silva SJR da, Kohl A, Pena L, et al. Recent insights into SARS-CoV-2 omicron variant. Reviews in Medical Virology 2023;**33**(1):e2373. DOI: 10.1002/rmv.2373

[17] outbreak.info SARS-CoV-2 data explorer. Availanle from: https://outbreak.info/ [Accessed: June 11, 2023]

[18] Xu A, Hong B, Lou F, et al. Sub-lineages of the SARS-CoV-2 Omicron variants: Characteristics and prevention. MedComm (2020). 2022;**3**(3):e172. DOI: 10.1002/mco2.172

[19] Scott L, Hsiao N, Moyo S, et al. Track Omicron's spread with molecular data. Science. 2021;**374**(6574):1454-1455. DOI: 10.1126/science.abn4543

[20] Torjesen I. Covid-19: Omicron may be more transmissible than other variants and partly resistant to existing vaccines, scientists fear. BMJ. 2021;**375**:n2943. DOI: 10.1136/bmj.n2943

[21] He X, Hong W, Pan X, et al. SARS-CoV-2 Omicron variant: Characteristics and prevention. MedComm (2020). 2021;**2**(4):838-845. DOI: 10.1002/mco2.110

[22] Karim SSA, Karim QA. Omicron SARS-CoV-2 variant: A new chapter in the COVID-19 pandemic. Lancet. 2021;**398**(10317):2126-2128. DOI: 10.1016/S0140-6736(21)02758-6

[23] Chatterjee S, Bhattacharya M, Nag S, et al. A detailed overview of SARS-CoV-2 omicron: Its sub-variants, mutations and pathophysiology, clinical characteristics, immunological landscape, immune escape, and therapies. Viruses. 2023;**15**(1):167. DOI: 10.3390/v15010167

[24] Gong SY, Chatterjee D, Richard J, et al. Contribution of single mutations to selected SARS-CoV-2 emerging variants spike antigenicity. Virology. 2021;**563**:134-145. DOI: 10.1016/j.virol.2021.09.001

[25] Wise J. Covid-19: The E484K mutation and the risks it poses. BMJ. 2021;**372**:n359. DOI: 10.1136/bmj.n359

[26] Zahradník J, Marciano S, Shemesh M, et al. SARS-CoV-2 variant prediction and antiviral drug design are enabled by RBD in vitro evolution. Nature Microbiology. 2021;**6**(9):1188-1198. DOI: 10.1038/s41564-021-00954-4

[27] Beyer DK, Forero A. Mechanisms of antiviral immune evasion of SARS-CoV-2. Journal of Molecular Biology. 2022;**434**(6):167265. DOI: 10.1016/j.jmb.2021.167265

[28] Thorne LG, Bouhaddou M, Reuschl A-K, et al. Evolution of enhanced innate immune evasion by the SARS-CoV-2 B.1.1.7 UK variant. bioRxiv. 2021:2021.06.06.446826. DOI: 10.1101/2021.06.06.446826

[29] Wu J, Shi Y, Pan X, et al. SARS-CoV-2 ORF9b inhibits RIG-I-MAVS antiviral signaling by interrupting K63-linked ubiquitination of NEMO. Cell Reports. 2021;**34**(7):108761. DOI: 10.1016/j.celrep.2021.108761

[30] Leary S, Gaudieri S, Parker MD, et al. Generation of a novel SARS-CoV-2 subgenomic RNA due to the R203K/G204R variant in nucleocapsid: Homologous recombination has potential to change SARS-CoV-2 at both protein and RNA level. bioRxiv. 2021:2020.04.10.029454. DOI: 10.1101/2020.04.10.029454

[31] Mourier T, Shuaib M, Hala S, et al. SARS-CoV-2 genomes from Saudi Arabia implicate nucleocapsid mutations in host response and increased viral load. Nature Communications. 2022;**13**(1):601. DOI: 10.1038/s41467-022-28287-8

[32] McMillen T, Jani K, Robilotti EV, et al. The spike gene target failure (SGTF) genomic signature is highly accurate for the identification of Alpha and Omicron SARS-CoV-2 variants. Scientific Reports. 2022;**12**(1):18968. DOI: 10.1038/s41598-022-21564-y

[33] Sarkar A, Omar S, Alshareef A, et al. The relative prevalence of the omicron variant within SARS-CoV-2 infected cohorts in different countries: A systematic review. Human Vaccines & Immunotherapeutics. 2023;**19**(1):2212568. DOI: 10.1080/21645515.2023.2212568

[34] Cao Y, Yisimayi A, Jian F, et al. BA.2.12.1, BA.4 and BA.5 escape antibodies elicited by Omicron infection. Nature. 2022;**608**(7923):593-602. DOI: 10.1038/s41586-022-04980-y

[35] Yamasoba D, Kimura I, Kosugi Y, et al. Neutralization sensitivity of Omicron BA.2.75 to therapeutic monoclonal antibodies. bioRxiv:2022.07.14.500041. DOI: 10.1101/2022.07.14.500041

[36] Cao Y, Song W, Wang L, et al. Characterization of the enhanced infectivity and antibody evasion of Omicron BA.2.75. Cell Host Microbe. 2022;**30**(11):1527-1539.e5. DOI: 10.1016/j.chom.2022.09.018

[37] Sheward DJ, Kim C, Fischbach J, et al. Evasion of neutralizing antibodies by Omicron sublineage BA.2.75. The Lancet Infectious Diseases. 2022;**22**(10):1421-1422. DOI: 10.1016/S1473-3099(22)00524-2

[38] Planas D, Bruel T, Staropoli I, et al. Resistance of Omicron subvariants BA.2.75.2, BA.4.6, and BQ.1.1 to neutralizing antibodies. bioRxiv. 2022:2022.11.17.516888. DOI: 10.1101/2022.11.17.516888

[39] Cao Y, Jian F, Wang J, et al. Imprinted SARS-CoV-2 humoral immunity induces convergent Omicron RBD evolution. Nature. 2023;**614**(7948):521-529. DOI: 10.1038/s41586-022-05644-7

[40] Kaku CI, Starr TN, Zhou P, et al. Evolution of antibody immunity following Omicron BA.1 breakthrough infection. Nature Communications. 2023;**14**(1):2751. DOI: 10.1038/s41467-023-38345-4

[41] Qu P, Evans JP, Faraone J, et al. Distinct neutralizing antibody escape of SARS-CoV-2 Omicron subvariants BQ.1, BQ.1.1, BA.4.6, BF.7 and BA.2.75.2. bioRxiv. 2022:2022.10.19.512891. DOI: 10.1101/2022.10.19.512891

[42] Mallapaty S. Can China avoid a wave of deaths if it lifts strict zero COVID policy? Nature. 2022;**612**(7939):203. DOI: 10.1038/d41586-022-04235-w

[43] Chenchula S, Amerneni KC, Ghanta MK, et al. Clinical virology and effect of Covid-19 vaccination and monoclonal antibodies against highly infectious SARS-CoV-2 omicron sub variant BF.7 (BA.5.2.1.7): A systematic review. Virology. 2023;**584**:38-43. DOI: 10.1016/j.virol.2023.04.007

[44] Yue C, Song W, Wang L, et al. ACE2 binding and antibody evasion in enhanced transmissibility of XBB.1.5. The Lancet Infectious Diseases. 2023;**23**(3):278-280. DOI: 10.1016/S1473-3099(23)00010-5

[45] Qu P, Faraone JN, Evans JP, et al. Extraordinary evasion of neutralizing antibody response by Omicron XBB.1.5, CH.1.1 and CA.3.1 variants. bioRxiv. 2023:2023.01.16.524244. DOI: 10.1101/2023.01.16.524244

[46] Lasrado N, Collier A-RY, Miller J, et al. Waning immunity against XBB.1.5 following bivalent mRNA boosters. bioRxiv. 2023:2023.01.22.525079. DOI: 10.1101/2023.01.22.525079

[47] Yamasoba D, Uriu K, Plianchaisuk A, et al. Virological characteristics of the SARS-CoV-2 Omicron XBB.1.16 variant. The Lancet Infectious Diseases. 2023;**23**(6):655-656. DOI: 10.1016/S1473-3099(23)00278-5

[48] Vashishtha VM, Kumar P. Preliminary clinical characteristics of Pediatric Covid-19 cases during the ongoing Omicron XBB.1.16 driven surge in a north Indian city. medRxiv:2023.04.18.23288715, 10.1101/2023.04.18.23288715

[49] World Health Organization. XBB.1.16 Initial Risk Assessment. 17 April 2023. Available from: https://www.who.int/docs/default-source/coronaviruse/21042023xbb.1.16ra-v2.pdf?sfvrsn=84577350_1

[50] Khera R, Jain S, Lin Z, et al. Evaluation of the anticipated burden of COVID-19 on hospital-based healthcare services across the United States. medRxiv. 2020:2020.04.01.20050492. DOI: 10.1101/2020.04.01.20050492

[51] Mogharab V, Ostovar M, Ruszkowski J, et al. Global burden of the COVID-19 associated patient-related delay in emergency healthcare: A panel of systematic review and meta-analyses. Globalization and Health. 2022;**18**(1):58. DOI: 10.1186/s12992-022-00836-2

[52] Bálint G, Vörös-Horváth B, Széchenyi A. Omicron: Increased transmissibility and decreased pathogenicity. Signal Transduction and Targeted Therapy. 2022;**7**(1):151. DOI: 10.1038/s41392-022-01009-8

[53] Alemi F, Vang J, Wojtusiak J, et al. Differential diagnosis of COVID-19 and influenza. PLOS Global Public Health. 2022;**2**(7):e0000221. DOI: 10.1371/journal.pgph.0000221

[54] Garrett N, Tapley A, Andriesen J, et al. High rate of asymptomatic carriage associated with variant strain Omicron. medRxiv. 2022:2021.12.20.21268130. DOI: 10.1101/2021.12.20.21268130

[55] Lewnard JA, Hong VX, Patel MM, et al. Clinical outcomes associated with SARS-CoV-2 Omicron (B.1.1.529) variant and BA.1/BA.1.1 or BA.2 subvariant infection in Southern California. Nature Medicine. 2022;**28**(9):1933-1943. DOI: 10.1038/s41591-022-01887-z

[56] Hui KPY, Ho JCW, Cheung MC, et al. SARS-CoV-2 omicron variant replication in human bronchus and lung ex vivo. Nature. 2022;**603**(7902):715-720. DOI: 10.1038/s41586-022-04479-6

[57] Lamers MM, Mykytyn AZ, Breugem TI, et al. SARS-CoV-2 Omicron efficiently infects human airway, but not alveolar epithelium. bioRxiv:2022.01.19.476898. DOI: 10.1101/2022.01.19.476898

[58] Arabi M, Al-Najjar Y, Mhaimeed N, et al. Severity of the Omicron SARS-CoV-2 variant compared with the previous lineages: A systematic

review. Journal of Cellular and Molecular Medicine;**27**(11):1443-1464. DOI: 10.1111/jcmm.17747

[59] Stowe J, Andrews N, Kirsebom F, et al. Effectiveness of COVID-19 vaccines against omicron and Delta hospitalisation, a test negative case-control study. Nature Communications. 2022;**13**(1):5736. DOI: 10.1038/s41467-022-33378-7

[60] Buchan SA, Chung H, Brown KA, et al. Estimated effectiveness of COVID-19 vaccines against omicron or Delta symptomatic infection and severe outcomes. JAMA Network Open. 2022;**5**(9):e2232760. DOI: 10.1001/jamanetworkopen.2022.32760

[61] Hyams C, Challen R, Marlow R, et al. Severity of Omicron (B.1.1.529) and Delta (B.1.617.2) SARS-CoV-2 infection among hospitalised adults: A prospective cohort study in Bristol, United Kingdom. Lancet Regional Health – Europe. 2023;**25**:100556. DOI: 10.1016/j.lanepe.2022.100556

[62] Kahn F, Bonander C, Moghaddassi M, et al. Risk of severe COVID-19 from the Delta and Omicron variants in relation to vaccination status, sex, age and comorbidities—Surveillance results from southern Sweden, July 2021 to January 2022. Euro Surveillance: European Communicable Disease Bulletin. 2022;**27**(9):2200121. DOI: 10.2807/1560-7917.ES.2022.27.9.2200121

[63] Sigal A, Milo R, Jassat W. Estimating disease severity of omicron and Delta SARS-CoV-2 infections. Nature Reviews. Immunology. 2022;**22**(5):267-269. DOI: 10.1038/s41577-022-00720-5

[64] Nyberg T, Ferguson NM, Nash SG, et al. Comparative analysis of the risks of hospitalisation and death associated with SARS-CoV-2 omicron (B.1.1.529) and delta (B.1.617.2) variants in England: A cohort study. Lancet. 2022;**399**(10332):1303-1312. DOI: 10.1016/S0140-6736(22)00462-7

[65] Ward IL, Bermingham C, Ayoubkhani D, et al. Risk of covid-19 related deaths for SARS-CoV-2 omicron (B.1.1.529) compared with delta (B.1.617.2): Retrospective cohort study. BMJ. 2022;**378**:e070695. DOI: 10.1136/bmj-2022-070695

[66] Khan A, Khan SA, Zia K, et al. Deciphering the impact of mutations on the binding efficacy of SARS-CoV-2 Omicron and Delta variants with human ACE2 receptor. Frontiers in Chemistry. 2022;**10**:892093. DOI: 10.3389/fchem.2022.892093

[67] Willett BJ, Grove J, MacLean OA, et al. SARS-CoV-2 omicron is an immune escape variant with an altered cell entry pathway. Nature Microbiology. 2022;**7**(8):1161-1179. DOI: 10.1038/s41564-022-01143-7

[68] Hachmann NP, Miller J, Collier AY, et al. Neutralization escape by SARS-CoV-2 Omicron subvariant BA.4.6. The New England Journal of Medicine. 2022;**387**(20):1904-1906. DOI: 10.1056/NEJMc2212117

[69] Qu P, Evans JP, Zheng YM, et al. Evasion of neutralizing antibody responses by the SARS-CoV-2 BA.2.75 variant. Cell Host Microbe. 2022;**30**(11):1518-1526.e4. DOI: 10.1016/j.chom.2022.09.015

[70] Qu P, Evans JP, Faraone JN, et al. Enhanced neutralization resistance of SARS-CoV-2 Omicron subvariants BQ.1, BQ.1.1, BA.4.6, BF.7, and BA.2.75.2. Cell Host Microbe. 2023;**31**(1):9-17.e3. DOI: 10.1016/j.chom.2022.11.012

[71] Pérez-Then E, Lucas C, Monteiro VS, et al. Neutralizing antibodies against the

SARS-CoV-2 Delta and Omicron variants following heterologous CoronaVac plus BNT162b2 booster vaccination. Nature Medicine. 2022;**28**(3):481-485. DOI: 10.1038/s41591-022-01705-6

[72] Rössler A, Riepler L, Bante D, et al. SARS-CoV-2 omicron variant neutralization in serum from vaccinated and convalescent persons. The New England Journal of Medicine. 2022;**386**(7):698-700. DOI: 10.1056/NEJMc2119236

[73] Accorsi EK, Britton A, Fleming-Dutra KE, et al. Association between 3 doses of mRNA COVID-19 vaccine and symptomatic infection caused by the SARS-CoV-2 Omicron and Delta variants. Journal of the American Medical Association. 2022;**327**(7):639-651. DOI: 10.1001/jama.2022.0470

[74] Lee HK, Knabl L, Moliva JI, et al. mRNA vaccination in octogenarians 15 and 20 months after recovery from COVID-19 elicits robust immune and antibody responses that include Omicron. Cell Reports. 2022;**39**(2):110680. DOI: 10.1016/j.celrep.2022.110680

[75] Garcia-Beltran WF, St. Denis KJ, Hoelzemer A, et al. mRNA-based COVID-19 vaccine boosters induce neutralizing immunity against SARS-CoV-2 Omicron variant. Cell. 2022;**185**(3):457-466.e4. DOI: 10.1016/j.cell.2021.12.033

[76] Lau JJ, Cheng SMS, Leung K, et al. Real-world COVID-19 vaccine effectiveness against the Omicron BA.2 variant in a SARS-CoV-2 infection-naive population. Nature Medicine. 2023;**29**(2):348-357. DOI: 10.1038/s41591-023-02219-5

[77] Chalkias S, Harper C, Vrbicky K, et al. A bivalent omicron-containing booster vaccine against Covid-19. The New England Journal of Medicine. 2022;**387**(14):1279-1291. DOI: 10.1056/NEJMoa2208343

[78] Caillard S, Thaunat O. COVID-19 vaccination in kidney transplant recipients. Nature Reviews. Nephrology. 2021;**17**(12):785-787. DOI: 10.1038/s41581-021-00491-7

[79] Haldane V, Jung AS, De Foo C, et al. Strengthening the basics: Public health responses to prevent the next pandemic. BMJ. 2021;**375**:e067510. DOI: 10.1136/bmj-2021-067510

[80] World Health Organization. Enhancing Response to Omicron SARS-CoV-2 Variant: Technical Brief and Priority Actions for Member States. 2022. Available from: https://www.who.int/publications/m/item/enhancing-readiness-for-omicron-(b.1.1.529)-technical-brief-and-priority-actions-for-member-states

[81] Hossain MJ, Rahman SMA, Emran TB, et al. Recommendation and roadmap of mass vaccination against coronavirus disease 2019 pandemic in Bangladesh as a lower-middle-income country. Archives of Razi Institute. 2021;**76**(6):1823-1830. DOI: 10.22092/ari.2021.356357.1824

[82] Salimi-Jeda A, Abbassi S, Mousavizadeh A, et al. SARS-CoV-2: Current trends in emerging variants, pathogenesis, immune responses, potential therapeutic, and vaccine development strategies. International Immunopharmacology. 2021;**101**(Pt A):108232. DOI: 10.1016/j.intimp.2021.108232

[83] Brito AF, Semenova E, Dudas G, et al. Global disparities in SARS-CoV-2 genomic surveillance. Nature Communications. 2022;**13**(1):7003. DOI: 10.1038/s41467-022-33713-y

[84] Hossain MJ, Soma MA, Islam MR, et al. Urgent call for actionable measures

to fight the current co-epidemic of dengue burden during the SARS-CoV-2 delta variant era in South-Asia. Ethics, Medicine, and Public Health. 2021;**19**:100726. DOI: 10.1016/j.jemep.2021.100726

[85] Asrani P, Tiwari K, Eapen MS, et al. Containment strategies for COVID-19 in India: Lessons from the second wave. Expert Review of Anti-Infective Therapy. 2022;**20**(6):829-835. DOI: 10.1080/14787210.2022.2036605

[86] Wahid M, Jawed A, Mandal RK, et al. Variants of SARS-CoV-2, their effects on infection, transmission and neutralization by vaccine induced antibodies. European Review for Medical and Pharmacological Sciences. 2021;**25**(18):5857-5864. DOI: 10.26355/eurrev_202109_26805

[87] Tareq AM, Emran TB, Dhama K, et al. Impact of SARS-CoV-2 delta variant (B.1.617.2) in surging second wave of COVID-19 and efficacy of vaccines in tackling the ongoing pandemic. Human Vaccines & Immunotherapeutics. 2021;**17**(11):4126-4127. DOI: 10.1080/21645515.2021.1963601

[88] Fiolet T, Kherabi Y, MacDonald C-J, et al. Comparing COVID-19 vaccines for their characteristics, efficacy and effectiveness against SARS-CoV-2 and variants of concern: A narrative review. Clinical Microbiology and Infection. 2022;**28**(2):202-221. DOI: 10.1016/j.cmi.2021.10.005

[89] Somerville M, Curran JA, Dol J, et al. Public health implications of SARS-CoV-2 variants of concern: A rapid scoping review. BMJ Open. 2021;**11**(12):e055781. DOI: 10.1136/bmjopen-2021-055781

[90] Redwan EM. COVID-19 pandemic and vaccination build herd immunity. European Review for Medical and Pharmacological Sciences. 2021;**25**(2):577-579. DOI: 10.26355/eurrev_202101_24613

[91] Dhama K, Nainu F, Frediansyah A, et al. Global emerging Omicron variant of SARS-CoV-2: Impacts, challenges and strategies. Journal of Infection and Public Health. 2023;**16**(1):4-14. DOI: 10.1016/j.jiph.2022.11.024

Chapter 5

Virulence and Infectivity Were Associated with Different Fragments in the Delta Subtype of SARS-CoV-2

Peijun Zuo, Longlong Zuo, Zhihong Li and Liping Li

Abstract

Since 2019, the antigens from Severe Acute Respiratory Syndrome Corona Virus 2 (SARS-CoV-2) have evolved from the initial D614 wild strain in the first epidemic wave, to D614G mutant in the second wave, to Delta mutant in the third wave, and to Omicron mutant in the fourth wave. Were the virulence and infectivity associated with different fragments in the Delta subtype of SARS-CoV-2? It is needed to analyze the sequences of the virus. The longest four glycine-free antigen fragments with tryptophan, longer or equal to 37 amino acids in length, were selected. The four fragment sequences in D614, D614G, N148, and I358 Omicron subtype were searched from the National Center of Biological Information website. The standard deviation (SD) of the molecular weight of the contained amino acids in the fragments was calculated to be the indicator of their antigen precession. The longest fragment was analyzed for the relationship between antigen precession and virus infectivity. On the other hand, 10 mutations in the Delta subtype were found in eight mutated fragments, and their antigen precession was used to analyze the correlation with virus virulence. The longest antigen fragments determined virus infectivity. Whole mutated fragments determined the virulence. Both were associated with different mutated fragments with varied antigen precession in the Delta subtype of SARS-CoV-2.

Keywords: antigen, evolution, D614, Delta, SARS-CoV-2

1. Introduction

In December 2019, coronavirus disease (COVID-19), with the unmutated D614 antigen, was first reported in China [1]. The epidemic, originating in Wuhan, China, started on December 12, 2019, causing 2794 laboratory-confirmed infections, and by January 26, 2020, these infections had resulted in 80 deaths.

On March 1, 2020, only 9.9% of the analyzed 6244 global cases were the second generation strain of SARS-Cov-2, referred to as D614G, but this rapidly increased to 54% by March 10, 2020, causing D614G to become the dominant strain [2]. Based on the D614 to D614G mutation, D614G, the Delta subtype, was mutated before

Omicron emerged, and there were 10 major mutated subtypes of SARS-CoV-2 [3]. These subtypes are shown in **Table 1**, and D614G is shown in bold. The SARS-Cov-2 B.1.617 lineage was found in India first [4] but quickly spread to other countries. The lineage includes three main subtypes: B1.617.1 (Kappa), B.1.617.2 (Delta), and B.617.3 (None-typed).

B.1.617.2 (Delta) first emerged in India in October 2020 [5]. As shown in **Table 1**, there were 10 common mutations, with some authors reporting five more noncommon, giving a total number of 15 mutations for Delta emerged before Omicron. The Omicron had at least 30 mutations.

The third generation of SARS-CoV-2 should be the Delta subtype. It is believed to have been transmitted faster than any other subtype, except for Omicron. Compared with the Alpha subtype (B.1.1.7), the sera collected from SARS-CoV-2 patients were fourfold less powerful against the Delta subtype [6]. Some authors considered that the antigenicity changes in the Delta subtype might not be sufficient against the current vaccines. In another paper the same team published, they compared the antigenicity with the H3N2 flu vaccine [7], suggesting that this may be the worst vaccine. But the truth was that most patients of the Delta subtype were immunized with the vaccine. We need to know why the vaccines did not work for the Delta subtype and also need to identify good vaccines.

The mutations occur and need to avoid the protective effects of vaccines. They also increased the limit of the detection. For example, the detection limit for the wild type D614 SARS-CoV-2 was 21.5 copies; for Omicron, it was 14.3 copies, but for the Delta subtype, it raised 32.0 copies [8]. The order for detection limitation was very similar to the order of virulence: Omicron was weakest, then D614, D614G, and Delta. Not all

Pango Linage	Origin	Subtypes	Spike mutations
B.1.1.7	UK	Alpha	H69del, V70del, E484K, S494P, N570D, **D614G**, P681H, T716I, S982A, K1191N
B.1.351	S. Africa	Beta	D80A, D215G, L241del, L242del, A243del, K417N, E484K, N501Y, **D614G**, A701V
P.1	Brazil/ Japan	Gamma	L18F, T20N, P26S, D138Y, R190S, K417T, E484K, N501Y, **D614G**, H655Y, T1027I
B.1.617.2	India	Delta	T19R, V70F*, T95I*, G142D, E156del, F157del, R158G, A222V*, W258L*, K417N*, L452R, T478K, **D614G**, P681R, D950N
B.1.427/ B.1.429	US	Epsilon	S13I, W152C, L452R, **D614G**
P.2	Brazil	Zeta	E484K, F565L, **D614G**, V1176F
B.1.525	UK/ Nigeria	Eta	A67V, H69del, V70del, E484K, **D614G**, Q677H, Q677H, F888L
B.1.526	US	Iota	L5F, D80G, T95I, Y144del, F157S, D253G, L452R, S477N, E484K, **D614G**, A701V, T859N, D950H, Q957R
B.1.617.1	India	Kappa	T95I, G142D, E154K, L452R, E484Q, **D614G**, P681R, Q1071H
B.1.617.3	India	None	T19R, G142D, L452R, E484Q, **D614G**, P681R, D950N

**Detected in some sequences but not all.*

Table 1.
Subtypes of SARS-CoV-2 mutants based on D614G.

patients of SARS-CoV-2 reached the detection limit, with the positive ratio of patients being as low as 47.21% [9]. Therefore, it is important to find the mutation route of SARS-CoV-2.

Some scientists try to find the regulation or rule for Delta and Delta plus mutations [10]. The authors analyzed the frequencies of the mutations, and the data set was numerous.

Some scientists use "deep phylogenetic-based clustering analysis" to uncover new and shared mutations in SARS-CoV-2 variants due to directional and convergent evolution [11]. The phylogenetic clustering analysis needs at least three sequences.

Two main Receptor-Binding Domain (RBD) conformations have been described, standing-up and lying-down states, with high and low affinity to ACE2, respectively [12, 13]. The standing-up and lying-down states are also qualified data.

However, our approach is different from other authors. We analyzed the trends of the "precession" changing in the mutated fragments, and the data were quantified. Our "precession" method can be analyzed as less than two sequences.

In the four waves of SARS-CoV-2, there were four main subtypes: D614, D614G, Delta, and Omicron. What caused such step-by-step evolutions of these four subtypes? In our previous work, we found the antigens of the SARS-CoV-2 showed a preference to evolve from most "rough" status and in a dose-dependent manner [14]. In the first two waves of SARS-CoV-2, the status of D614, caused by the first wave, was "rough"; meanwhile, the status of D614G, caused by the second wave, was "precise".

Besides D614G, did the other nine confirmed mutations in the Delta type follow the same trend as D614G, from "rough" to "precise", after mutation? We analyzed data to confirm if this way was true in this paper.

This paper will try to find a regulation or a rule for the longest fragments, longer or equal to 37 amino acids in length if the mutants first happened in the position of "rough", but not in other positions. If the infectivity is associated with the longest fragments. We will also examine if, after mutation, the "rough" status of mutants in the Delta type was changed to "precise" in the fragments of N148 (E156del, F157del, and R158G), T19R, G142D, L452R, T478K, D614G, P681R, and D950N. If the precession of the whole mutation is associated with the virulence.

2. Materials and methods

2.1 Access protein sequences

At the website https://www.ncbi.nlm.nih.gov/, select Protein in All Databases. Put the access number to search the protein sequence of the subtype SARS-CoV-2.

The amino acid sequence of protein "QHD43416" containing D614, and the sequences of protein "7KDK_A", "7V8A_B", and "7V8A_C" containing D614G.

The amino acid sequences of proteins "7V8B_A", "7V8A_B", and "7V8A_C" contained the Delta subtypes, with mutations of N148 (E156del, F157del, and R158G), T19R, G142D, L452R, T478K, D614G, P681R, and D950N.

2.2 Alignment protein sequences of the subtype SARS-CoV-2

At the website, https://www.ebi.ac.uk/Tools/msa/clustalo/, select Protein at the Enter or paste a set of.

Input the protein sequences of SARS-CoV-2 original sequence, D614, the D614G mutants, and the Delta subtype and Submit.

In the alignment result of Clustal Omega, all "G" amino acids were shown in yellow (**Figures 1–4**).

2.3 Select longest G-free antigen fragments longer or equal to 37 amino acids in length

In the original D614 subtype of SARS-CoV-2, QHD43416, select the G-free antigen fragments longer or equal to 37 amino acids. Such fragments do not contain any G, glycine. Normally, the non-G amino acid has the mutation potential to a smaller amino acid. Glycine is the smallest amino acid. The selected results are shown in **Table 2**.

2.4 Find whole mutation fragment in Delta subtype of SARS-CoV-2

In sequence of Delta subtype of SARS-CoV-2, "7V8B_A", "7V8A_B", and "7V8A_C", find the mutations of N148 (E156del, F157del, R158G), T19R, G142D, L452R, T478K, D614G, P681R, and D950N. The fragments may contain G amino acid, but the least rough fragments were selected. The results are shown in **Table 3**. The mutations contain eight fragments and 10 site mutations in the Delta subtype. These eight fragments were compared and shown in **Figure 5**.

2.5 Calculate the precession of whole mutation fragment in Delta subtype of SARS-CoV-2

In each fragment, the molecular weight of contained amino acid were different. The mean and standard deviations (SD) of molecular weight were calculated using Excel. The results are shown in **Tables 2** and **3**. The standard deviations (SD) of molecular weight can indicate precession. The smaller the SD, the rougher the precession, and the easier it is to be recognized by the immune system. The fragment precession was calculated both before and after the mutation.

3. Results

3.1 The longest G-free peptide with Tryptophan (W) longer or equal to 37 amino acids in length

3.1.1 The antigen fragment D614 in the original strain, led the first wave of epidemic

As shown in **Table 2**, the D614 peptide has a mean molecular weight of 129.3, and the standard deviation (SD) for the individual molecular weight of its amino acids is 25.23. This peptide contains the biggest amino acid, tryptophan (W, molecular weight, 204.2262). In the "W" contained fragments, the SD of D614, 25.23 was the smallest among the G-free peptides. This means that the status is the "roughest" and that this location is the most likely place for a mutation. This site has already been confirmed to have the D614G mutation.

As shown in **Figure 2**, the candidates of mutant peptides are the arrowed fragments. The first is D614, TNTSNQVAVLYQDVNCTEVPVAIHADQLTPTWRVYST, 37 amino acids in length. This G-free fragment contains the D614 amino acid in the

```
                                                     F58→→→→→→→→→→
QHD43416    MFVFLVLLPLVSSQCVNLTTRTQLPPAYTNSFTRGVYYPDKVFRSSVLHSTQDLFLPFFS    60
7V8B_A      mfvflvllplvssqcvnlrtrtqlppaytnsftrgvyypdkvfrssvlhstqdlflpffs    60
7V8A_B      mfvflvllplvssqcvnlrtrtqlppaytnsftrgvyypdkvfrssvlhstqdlflpffs    60
7V8A_C      mfvflvllplvssqcvnlrtrtqlppaytnsftrgvyypdkvfrssvlhstqdlflpffs    60
7KDK_A      mfvflvllplvssqcvnlttrtqlppaytnsftrgvyypdkvfrssvlhstqdlflpffs    60
            ****************** *****************************************
       F58→→→→
QHD43416    NVTWFHAIHVSGTNGTKRFDNPVLPFNDGVYFASTEKSNIIRGWIFGTTLDSKTQSLLIV    120
7V8B_A      nvtwfhaihvsgtngtkrfdnpvlpfndgvyfasteksniirgwifgttldsktqslliv    120
7V8A_B      nvtwfhaihvsgtngtkrfdnpvlpfndgvyfasteksniirgwifgttldsktqslliv    120
7V8A_C      nvtwfhaihvsgtngtkrfdnpvlpfndgvyfasteksniirgwifgttldsktqslliv    120
7KDK_A      nvtwfhaihvsgtngtkrfdnpvlpfndgvyfasteksniirgwifgttldsktqslliv    120
            ************************************************************
                                N148→→→→→→→→→→→→→→→→→→→
                              G142D→→→→→→
QHD43416    NNATNVVIKVCEFQFCNDPFLGVYYHKNNKSWMESEFRVYSSANNCTFEYVSQPFLMDLE    180
7V8B_A      nnatnvvikvcefqfcndpfldvyyhknnkswmes--gvyssannctfeyvsqpflmdle    178
7V8A_B      nnatnvvikvcefqfcndpfldvyyhknnkswmes--gvyssannctfeyvsqpflmdle    178
7V8A_C      nnatnvvikvcefqfcndpfldvyyhknnkswmes--gvyssannctfeyvsqpflmdle    178
7KDK_A      nnatnvvikvcefqfcndpflgvyyhknnkswmesefrvyssannctfeyvsqpflmdle    180
            *********************.*************   **********************

QHD43416    GKQGNFKNLREFVFKNIDGYFKIYSKHTPINLVRDLPQGFSALEPLVDLPIGINITRFQT    240
7V8B_A      gkqgnfknlrefvfknidgyfkiyskhtpinlvrdlpqgfsaleplvdlpiginitrfqt    238
7V8A_B      gkqgnfknlrefvfknidgyfkiyskhtpinlvrdlpqgfsaleplvdlpiginitrfqt    238
7V8A_C      gkqgnfknlrefvfknidgyfkiyskhtpinlvrdlpqgfsaleplvdlpiginitrfqt    238
7KDK_A      gkqgnfknlrefvfknidgyfkiyskhtpinlvrdlpqgfsaleplvdlpiginitrfqt    240
            ************************************************************

QHD43416    LLALHRSYLTPGDSSSGWTAGAAAYYVGYLQPRTFLLKYNENGTITDAVDCALDPLSETK    300
7V8B_A      llalhrsyltpgdsssgwtagaaayyvgylqprtfllkynengtitdavdcaldplsetk    298
7V8A_B      llalhrsyltpgdsssgwtagaaayyvgylqprtfllkynengtitdavdcaldplsetk    298
7V8A_C      llalhrsyltpgdsssgwtagaaayyvgylqprtfllkynengtitdavdcaldplsetk    298
7KDK_A      llalhrsyltpgdsssgwtagaaayyvgylqprtfllkynengtitdavdcaldplsetk    300
            ************************************************************
```

Figure 1.
The amino acids of N148 and G142D. The amino acid sequence of protein "QHD43416" contained D614, "7KDK_A", contained G614, "7V8B_A", "7V8A_B", "7V8A_C" contained Delta subtype were searched from NCBI. The amino acid sequences of D614, the G614 mutant, and Delta subtype were compared with the online software of Clustal Omega. In the alignment result of Clustal Omega, all "G" amino acids are marked by the yellow color. N148 and G142D were indicated by the arrows.

```
                                                I358→→→→→→→→→→
QHD43416    CTLKSFTVEKGIYQTSNFRVQPTESIVRFPNITNLCPFGEVFNATRFASVYAWNRKRISN    360
7V8B_A      ctlksftvekgiyqtsnfrvqptesivrfpnitnlcpfgevfnatrfasvyawnrkrisn    358
7V8A_B      ctlksftvekgiyqtsnfrvqptesivrfpnitnlcpfgevfnatrfasvyawnrkrisn    358
7V8A_C      ctlksftvekgiyqtsnfrvqptesivrfpnitnlcpfgevfnatrfasvyawnrkrisn    358
7KDK_A      ctlksftvekgiyqtsnfrvqptesivrfpnitnlcpfgevfnatrfasvyawnrkrisn    360
            ************************************************************
      I358→→→→→→→→→→
QHD43416    CVADYSVLYNSASFSTFKCYGVSPTKLNDLCFTNVYADSFVIRGDEVRQIAPGQTGKIAD    420
7V8B_A      cvadysvlynsasfstfkcygvsptklndlcftnvyadsfvirgdevrqiapgqtgkiad    418
7V8A_B      cvadysvlynsasfstfkcygvsptklndlcftnvyadsfvirgdevrqiapgqtgkiad    418
7V8A_C      cvadysvlynsasfstfkcygvsptklndlcftnvyadsfvirgdevrqiapgqtgkiad    418
7KDK_A      cvadysvlynsasfstfkcygvsptklndlcftnvyadsfvirgdevrqiapgqtgkiad    420
            ************************************************************
                                L452R→→→→→→→→→→→T478K
QHD43416    YNYKLPDDFTGCVIAWNSNNLDSKVGGNYNYLYRLFRKSNLKPFERDISTEIYQAGSTPC    480
7V8B_A      ynyklpddftgcviawnsnnldskvggnynyryrlfrksnlkpferdisteiyqagskpc    478
7V8A_B      ynyklpddftgcviawnsnnldskvggnynyryrlfrksnlkpferdisteiyqagskpc    478
7V8A_C      ynyklpddftgcviawnsnnldskvggnynyryrlfrksnlkpferdisteiyqagskpc    478
7KDK_A      ynyklpddftgcviawnsnnldskvggnynylyrlfrksnlkpferdisteiyqagstpc    480
            ****************************** **************************.**
      T478K
QHD43416    NGVEGFNCYFPLQSYGFQPTNGVGYQPYRVVVLSFELLHAPATVCGPKKSTNLVKNKCVN    540
7V8B_A      ngvegfncyfplqsygfqptngvgyqpyrvvvlsfellhapatvcgpkkstnlvknkcvn    538
7V8A_B      ngvegfncyfplqsygfqptngvgyqpyrvvvlsfellhapatvcgpkkstnlvknkcvn    538
7V8A_C      ngvegfncyfplqsygfqptngvgyqpyrvvvlsfellhapatvcgpkkstnlvknkcvn    538
7KDK_A      ngvegfncyfplqsygfqptngvgyqpyrvvvlsfellhapatvcgpkkstnlvknkcvn    540
            ************************************************************

QHD43416    FNFNGLTGTGVLTESNKKFLPFQQFGRDIADTTDAVRDPQTLEILDITPCSFGGVSVITP    600
7V8B_A      fnfngltgtgvltesnkkflpfqqfgrdiadttdavrdpqtleilditpcsfggvsvitp    598
7V8A_B      fnfngltgtgvltesnkkflpfqqfgrdiadttdavrdpqtleilditpcsfggvsvitp    598
7V8A_C      fnfngltgtgvltesnkkflpfqqfgrdiadttdavrdpqtleilditpcsfggvsvitp    598
7KDK_A      fnfngltgtgvltesnkkflpfqqfgrdiadttdavrdpqtleilditpcsfggvsvitp    600
            ************************************************************
         D614→→→→→→→→→→→→→→
QHD43416    GTNTSNQVAVLYQDVNCTEVPVAIHADQLTPTWRVYSTGSNVFQTRAGCLIGAEHVNNSY    660
7V8B_A      gtntsnqvavlyqgvnctevpvaihadqltptwrvystgsnvfqtragcligaehvnnsy    658
7V8A_B      gtntsnqvavlyqgvnctevpvaihadqltptwrvystgsnvfqtragcligaehvnnsy    658
7V8A_C      gtntsnqvavlyqgvnctevpvaihadqltptwrvystgsnvfqtragcligaehvnnsy    658
7KDK_A      gtntsnqvavlyqgvnctevpvaihadqltptwrvystgsnvfqtragcligaehvnnsy    660
            *************.**********************************************
```

Figure 2.
The amino acids of I358, L452R, T478K, and D614. In the alignment result of Clustal Omega, all "G" amino acids were marked by the yellow color. I358, L452R, and D614 were indicated by the arrows. I358 was mutated in the Omicron subtype.

```
                P681R→→→→→→→→→→→→→→F718→→→→→→→→
QHD43416    ECDIPIGAGICASYQTQTNSPRRARSVASQSIIAYTMSLGAENSVAYSNNSIAIPTNFTI    720
7V8B_A      ecdipigagicasyqtqtnsrgsassvasqsiiaytmslgaensvaysnnsiaiptnfti    718
7V8A_B      ecdipigagicasyqtqtnsrgsassvasqsiiaytmslgaensvaysnnsiaiptnfti    718
7V8A_C      ecdipigagicasyqtqtnsrgsassvasqsiiaytmslgaensvaysnnsiaiptnfti    718
7KDK_A      ecdipigagicasyqtqtnspgsassvasqsiiaytmslgaensvaysnnsiaiptnfti    720
            ********************   * ***********************************

        F718→→→→→→→→→
QHD43416    SVTTEILPVSMTKTSVDCTMYICGDSTECSNLLLQYGSFCTQLNRALTGIAVEQDKNTQE    780
7V8B_A      svtteilpvsmtktsvdctmyicgdstecsnlllqygsfctqlnraltgiaveqdkntqe    778
7V8A_B      svtteilpvsmtktsvdctmyicgdstecsnlllqygsfctqlnraltgiaveqdkntqe    778
7V8A_C      svtteilpvsmtktsvdctmyicgdstecsnlllqygsfctqlnraltgiaveqdkntqe    778
7KDK_A      svtteilpvsmtktsvdctmyicgdstecsnlllqygsfctqlnraltgiaveqdkntqe    780
            ************************************************************

QHD43416    VFAQVKQIYKTPPIKDFGGFNFSQILPDPSKPSKRSFIEDLLFNKVTLADAGFIKQYGDC    840
7V8B_A      vfaqvkqiyktppikdfggfnfsqilpdpskpskrsfiedllfnkvtladagfikqygdc    838
7V8A_B      vfaqvkqiyktppikdfggfnfsqilpdpskpskrsfiedllfnkvtladagfikqygdc    838
7V8A_C      vfaqvkqiyktppikdfggfnfsqilpdpskpskrsfiedllfnkvtladagfikqygdc    838
7KDK_A      vfaqvkqiyktppikdfggfnfsqilpdpskpskrsfiedllfnkvtladagfikqygdc    840
            ************************************************************

QHD43416    LGDIAARDLICAQKFNGLTVLPPLLTDEMIAQYTSALLAGTITSGWTFGAGAALQIPFAM    900
7V8B_A      lgdiaardlicaqkfngltvlpplltdemiaqytsallagtitsgwtfgagaalqipfam    898
7V8A_B      lgdiaardlicaqkfngltvlpplltdemiaqytsallagtitsgwtfgagaalqipfam    898
7V8A_C      lgdiaardlicaqkfngltvlpplltdemiaqytsallagtitsgwtfgagaalqipfam    898
7KDK_A      lgdiaardlicaqkfngltvlpplltdemiaqytsallagtitsgwtfgagaalqipfam    900
            ************************************************************
```

Figure 3.
The amino acids of P681R and F718. In the alignment result of Clustal Omega, all "G" amino acids were marked by the yellow color. P681R and F718 were indicated by the arrows.

original strain in Wuhan, China, on December 12, 2019, which led to the first wave of the epidemic. The precession of this fragment is 25.23, shown in **Table 2**.

3.1.2 The antigen fragment D614G in the Italian strain led to the second wave of epidemic

The D614 has already been confirmed as a mutated peptide. It mutated to D614G on March 10, 2020, first emerged in Italy, and led to the second wave of the epidemic. The precession of this fragment is increased to 26.74, shown in **Table 3**. This D614G mutation remains no change in D614G, Delta, and Omicron subtype. D614G has 37 amino acids, the molecular weight is 127.7, the SD is 26.74, and it contains "W".

```
                                                                     D950N→→→→→→→→
QHD43416    QMAYRFNGIGVTQNVLYENQKLIANQFNSAIGKIQDSLSSTASALGKLQDVVNQNAQALN    960
7V8B_A      qmayrfngigvtqnvlyenqklianqfnsaigkiqdslsstasalgklqnvvnqnaqaln    958
7V8A_B      qmayrfngigvtqnvlyenqklianqfnsaigkiqdslsstasalgklqnvvnqnaqaln    958
7V8A_C      qmayrfngigvtqnvlyenqklianqfnsaigkiqdslsstasalgklqnvvnqnaqaln    958
7KDK_A      qmayrfngigvtqnvlyenqklianqfnsaigkiqdslsstasalgklqdvvnqnaqaln    960
            *************************************************:**********

       D950N→→→→→                           I1018→→→→→→→→→→→→→→
QHD43416    TLVKQLSSNFGAISSVLNDILSRLDKVEAEVQIDRLITGRLQSLQTYVTQQLIRAAEIRA    1020
7V8B_A      tlvkqlssnfgaissvlndilsrldppeaevqidrlitgrlqslqtyvtqqliraaeira    1018
7V8A_B      tlvkqlssnfgaissvlndilsrldppeaevqidrlitgrlqslqtyvtqqliraaeira    1018
7V8A_C      tlvkqlssnfgaissvlndilsrldppeaevqidrlitgrlqslqtyvtqqliraaeira    1018
7KDK_A      tlvkqlssnfgaissvlndilsrldkveaevqidrlitgrlqslqtyvtqqliraaeira    1020
            *************************  *********************************

      I1018→→→→→→→→
QHD43416    SANLAATKMSECVLGQSKRVDFCGKGYHLMSFPQSAPHGVVFLHVTYVPAQEKNFTTAPA    1080
7V8B_A      sanlaatkmsecvlgqskrvdfcgkgyhlmsfpqsaphgvvflhvtyvpaqeknfttapa    1078
7V8A_B      sanlaatkmsecvlgqskrvdfcgkgyhlmsfpqsaphgvvflhvtyvpaqeknfttapa    1078
7V8A_C      sanlaatkmsecvlgqskrvdfcgkgyhlmsfpqsaphgvvflhvtyvpaqeknfttapa    1078
7KDK_A      sanlaatkmsecvlgqskrvdfcgkgyhlmsfpqsaphgvvflhvtyvpaqeknfttapa    1080
            ************************************************************

                                                               Y1138→→→→→
QHD43416    ICHDGKAHFPREGVFVSNGTHWFVTQRNFYEPQIITTDNTFVSGNCDVVIGIVNNTVYDP    1140
7V8B_A      ichdgkahfpregvfvsngthwfvtqrnfyepqiittdntfvsgncdvvigivnntvydp    1138
7V8A_B      ichdgkahfpregvfvsngthwfvtqrnfyepqiittdntfvsgncdvvigivnntvydp    1138
7V8A_C      ichdgkahfpregvfvsngthwfvtqrnfyepqiittdntfvsgncdvvigivnntvydp    1138
7KDK_A      ichdgkahfpregvfvsngthwfvtqrnfyepqiittdntfvsgncdvvigivnntvydp    1140
            ************************************************************

      Y1138→→→→→→→→→→→→→→
QHD43416    LQPELDSFKEELDKYFKNHTSPDVDLGDISGINASVVNIQKEIDRLNEVAKNLNESLIDL    1200
7V8B_A      lqpeldsfkeeldkyfknhtspdvdlgdisginasvvniqkeidrlnevaknlneslidl    1198
7V8A_B      lqpeldsfkeeldkyfknhtspdvdlgdisginasvvniqkeidrlnevaknlneslidl    1198
7V8A_C      lqpeldsfkeeldkyfknhtspdvdlgdisginasvvniqkeidrlnevaknlneslidl    1198
7KDK_A      lqpeldsfkeeldkyfknhtspdvdlgdisginasvvniqkeidrlnevaknlneslidl    1200
            ************************************************************

QHD43416    QELGKYEQYIKWPWYIWLGFIAGLIAI------VMVTIMLCCMTSCCSCLKGCCSCGSCC    1254
7V8B_A      qelgkyeqefgsggyipeaprdgqayvrkdgewvllstflkgqdnsa-diqh---sgrp-    1253
7V8A_B      qelgkyeqefgsggyipeaprdgqayvrkdgewvllstflkgqdnsa-diqh---sgrp-    1253
7V8A_C      qelgkyeqefgsggyipeaprdgqayvrkdgewvllstflkgqdnsa-diqh---sgrp-    1253
7KDK_A      qelgkyeqg---sgyipeaprdgqayvrkdgewvllstflgrslevl--fqg---pghhh    1252
            ********      **  .   *   :       *::: :*     .     ::     *
```

Figure 4.
The amino acids of D950N. In the alignment result of Clustal Omega, all "G" amino acids were marked by the yellow color. D950N was indicated by the arrow.

Peptides	Amino acids	Mean of molecular weight	SD	Contains "W"
F718	43	125.3	20.69	N
I358	41	134.2 (Omicron)	31.66(3)	Y
N148	38	140.1 (Delta)	26.92(2)	Y
D614	37	129.3 (D614G)	25.23(1)	Y

In the "W" contained fragments, among non-"G" peptides, the SD in D614, 25.23 is the smallest. This means the status is most "rough". Most likely, the mutation will happen to here. This is already confirmed by the G614 mutation. The N148 was the mutant confirmed by the Delta subtype, and the I358 was also a mutant confirmed by the Omicron subtype. The order was the evolution from "rough" to "precise". These antigens were also evolved to "precise" status.

Table 2.
The molecular weight and SD of D614, N148, I358, and another candidate of potential mutant peptide.

Peptides	Amino acids	Mean of molecular weight	SD	Contains "W"
T19	34	130.9	22.46	N
T19R	34	132.6	23.54↑	N
G142	17	144.9	32.31	Y
G142D	17	140.7	33.06↑	Y
N148	38	140.1	26.92	Y
E156del	36	136.5	28.65↑	Y
F157del	36	136.5	28.65↑	Y
R158G	36	136.5	28.65↑	Y
L452	28	143.9	25.86	N
L452R	28	145.4	26.35↑	N
T478	5	118.5	9.798	N
T478K	5	123.9	15.83↑	N
D614	37	129.3	25.23	Y
D614G	37	127.7	26.74↑	Y
P681	30	127.6	28.36	N
P681R	30	129.5	29.49↑	N
R682G	30	124.3	28.51↑	N
R683S	30	123.9	28.68↑	N
R685S	30	127.2	28.57↑	N
D950	24	128.6	18.64	N
D950N	24	128.6	18.64→	N

Beside 10 mutants N148 (E156del, F157del, R158G), T19R, G142D, L452R, T478K, D614G, P681R, D950N in Delta subtype, G682, S683, S685 were also mutants at least in "7V8B_A", "7V8A_B", "7V8A_C". Twelve in 13 were mutated from "rough" status to "precise"; only 1, D950N, was not changed.

Table 3.
The molecular weight and SD of D614, N148, and confirmed mutant peptides in Delta subtype.

```
D950    ----------------------KLQDVVNQNAQA-------LNTLVKQLSSNF------  24
G142    GVYYHKNNKSWMESEFR------------------------------------------  17
N148    -VYYHKNNKSWMESEFRVY----SSANNCTFEY---------------VSQPFLMDLE-  38
P681    ---------------------------ICASYQTQTNSPRRARSVASQSIIAYTMSL--  30
D614    -----TNTSNQVAVL--------YQDVNCTEVPVAIH--------ADQLTPTWRVYST-  37
L452    -------NYNYLYRLFRKSNLKPFERDIST--------------------EIYQA----  28
T19     --------------MFVFLVLLPLVSSQCVNLTT-----------RTQLPPAYTNSFTR  34
T478    -------------------------STPCN-----------------------------  5
```

Figure 5.
Eight fragments containing 10 confirmed mutations from the Delta subtype were selected. These fragments were compared.

3.1.3 The antigen fragment N148 in the Indian strain, led the third wave of epidemic

The other longer G-free peptide is N148, 38 amino acids in length, VYYHKNNKSWMESEFRVYSSANNCTFEYVSQPFLMDLE, as shown in **Figure 1**. This fragment has also already been confirmed as a mutated peptide in the Delta variant. It mutated in October 2020, in India and led to the third wave of epidemic. The precession of this fragment is 26.92 before mutation, larger than the precession of D614 and D614G, shown in **Table 2**. Its precession increased to 28.65 after the mutations on the same base as the D614G mutant (E156del, F157del, and R158G), shown in **Table 3**. N148 has 38 amino acids, the molecular weight is 140.1, the SD is 26.92, and it contains "W".

3.1.4 The antigen fragment I358 in the south African strain led the fourth wave of epidemic

Another identified peptide is I358, 41 amino acids in length, EVFNATRFAS-VYAWNRKRISNCVADYSVLYNSASFSTFKCY, as shown in **Figure 2**. I358 mutation confirmed by the Omicron subtype. The order of evolution was from "rough" to "precise", and these antigens were also shown to evolve to "precise" status.

The fragment was mutated on November 23, 2021, in South Africa, led to a fourth epidemic. The precession of this fragment is 31.66 before mutation, larger than the precession of D614, D614G, and Delta, as shown in **Tables 2** and **3**. The precession increased also. We will show the data in another paper. This peptide was also confirmed as an Omicron mutant. I358 has 41 amino acids, the molecular weight is 134.2, the SD is 31.66, and it contains "W".

3.2 The longest G-free peptide without Tryptophan, W

The longest G-free peptide without tryptophan, W, is F718, 43 amino acids in length, AENSVAYSNNSIAIPTNFTISVTTEILPVSMTKTSVDCTMYIC, as shown in **Figure 3**. F718 has 43 amino acids, the molecular weight is 125.3, the SD is 20.69, and it does not contain "W".

3.3 Whole mutated fragments in Delta subtypes D614G, N148 (E156del, F157del, and R158G), T19R, G142D, L452R, T478K, P681R, and D950N

Ten confirmed mutations observed in the Delta subtype are listed in **Table 1**. They are T19R, G142D, E156del, F157del, R158G, L452R, T478K, D614G, P681R, and

D950N (**Figure 4**). Their molecular weights and SDs are shown in **Table 3**. The data shown in green indicates the parameters of the antigens before mutation. All mutated antigens, after evolution, are shown in yellow. Their SDs were shown to have increased in nine of the confirmed mutations. Only 1 SD showed no change, but no SD was shown to have decreased.

Beside 10 mutants N148 (E156del, F157del, R158G), T19R, G142D, L452R, T478K, D614G, P681R, and D950N in the Delta subtype, G682, S683, and S685 were also mutants, at least in "7V8B_A", "7V8A_B", and "7V8A_C". Twelve of the 13 were mutated from "rough" status to "precise"; only one mutant, D950N, showed no change. At least 92.31% of the antigens had evolved from "rough" to "precise", and only 7.69% showed no change.

4. Discussion

4.1 The longest fragments of G-free and with W antigen longer or equal than 37 amino acid

4.1.1 First wave of COVID-19 caused by D614

COVID-19 was broken out in Wuhan, China, on December 12, 2019. The original strain was D614.

From the sequence of D614, the four longest fragments of G-free and with W antigen longer or equal to 37 amino acids was found. They were D614, N148, and I358.

Before COVID-19 went mutated, the D614, N148, and I358 existed independent from any mutation.

For proteins or antigens, the SD of the molecular weight can work as an indicator of its "fineness". The bigger the SD, the more the "fineness" or the more "precise" the protein or antigen is. In contrast, the smaller the SD, the "rougher" the protein or antigen is.

4.1.2 Second wave was caused by a mutation of D614 to D614G

The SD for D614 is 25.23. It is the smallest SD among the four longest antigens. It was mutated first on March 10, 2020. The mutated strain was D614G. The spike protein of SARS-CoV-2 contains about 1000 amino acids, and the D614 antigen contains only 37 amino acids. If this antigen mutated by chance, the possibility is only 3.7%, less than 5%, a small possibility. This mutation was not by chance, then by what?

The relationship between antigen and antibody is very similar to locker and key. A precision key can open any low-precision locker. The precision antibody should recognize and capture any low precession antibody. A precession key is a little smaller than the original key; otherwise, it cannot enter the space of the original locker. The D614G is a little smaller than D614 because G is the smallest amino acid.

Why did the mutation occur at D614 but not in the longer fragments, N148 or I358?

The virus would like to stay in the human body as long as possible. It would not to mutate the highest pressure status because the human body can generate the highest precision antibody to capture and neutralize it. If this were to happen, the virus could survive only 14 days in a single human body. The virus can stay in the human population for 3 months with the spread time.

The best way for the virus is to mutate to the next immediate degree. The D614G mutation proved this, and the precession was promoted from 25.23 to 26.74.

Therefore, the structure of D614G is the result of evolution, a more "precise" or complex status.

The human body has to generate more precession antibodies to recognize it.

The longest antigen, D614, worked as a factor to escape from the immune system; this is a factor to increase the infectivity of the virus.

4.1.3 Third wave was caused by mutation from D614G to Delta

The precession of D614G was promoted from 25.23 to 26.74. Which fragments will be mutated in the next immediate step?

The SD for N148 is 26.92 and the SD for I358 is 31.66. The virus would like to mutate the immediately next precision antigen, N148.

The third wave was caused by Delta subtype in October 2020 in India. N148 did mutate to a new antigen with three site mutations, E156del, F157del, and R158G, in this time and in the right order. The final precession was improved from 26.92 to 28.65. The size of the antigen was also decreased.

N148 is an antigen with 38 amino acids. If the mutation is mutated by chance, the single-site mutation rate is 3.8%, and if the three-site mutation happened in the N148 fragment, the mutation rate is 5.487×10^{-5}. It is an extremely small possibility and not mutated by chance. It did mutate after the second wave of D614G, also 10 months after the first wave broke out in Wuhan, China,

The possibility of D614 mutated D614G, then mutated to Delta is lower than 2.03×10^{-6}.

The longest antigens D614 and N148, worked as a factor to escape from the immune system; this is a factor to increase the infectivity of the virus.

4.1.4 Fourth wave was caused by mutation from Delta to Omicron

The precession of Delta was promoted from 26.92 to 28.65. Which fragments will be mutated in the next immediate step?

The SD for I358 is 31.66. This is the last choice for the virus to mutate in this antigen.

It did mutate on November 23, 2021, in the Omicron strain, leading to the fourth wave in South Africa.

The SD and the incubation time are shown to work in a dose-dependent manner. Such an effect is statistically significant, suggesting the order of evolution is correct and consistent with history. The D614G mutation happened first, the Delta subtype second, and the Omicron subtype third.

The I358 contains 41 amino acids. If the mutation happened by chance, the possibility was lower than 4.1% and a low possibility. It did not mutate by chance and mutated by the precession improvement. The possibility of D614 mutating to D614G, then mutating to Delta, then to Omicron is lower than 8.323×10^{-8}.

Although the antigen precession did not predict the epidemic of the Alpha, Beta, and Gama subtypes, the failure of the prediction did prove it is true. The Alpha, Beta, and Gama subtypes did not form the major wave in the world. There were no cases in China for the three subtypes. The antigen precession can only predict the major epidemic.

The longest antigens, D614, N148, and I 358, worked as a factor to escape from the immune system; this is a factor to increase the infectivity of the virus.

4.2 The longest fragments of G-free and without W antigen longer or equal to 37 amino acid

The F718 fragment has an SD of 20.69, which is even smaller than 25.23. Why did this "rough" fragment not mutate? The possible reason might be the distribution of the amino acids as it did not contain any of the biggest amino acids, tryptophan (W). If any peptide did not contain "W", it might not tend to be mutated in the first order.

To exclude the non-"W" fragments as potential candidates for evolution is a concern of statistical bias and could interfere with the SD calculations.

Tryptophan has its own biochemical functions, one being that it can be translated from a "stop codon". It is reported that the Thymine-Guanine-Adenine (TGA, stop) codon in Spiroplasma is for tryptophan instead of a stop signal in other species [15].

Tryptophan may play an important role in the infectivity. It needed to be studied further.

4.3 Whole mutated fragments determine the virulence

4.3.1 Whole mutation antigens in Delta subtype, D614G, N148 (E156del, F157del, R158G), T19R, G142D, L452R, T478K, P681R, D950N

In the 10 mutants of the Delta subtype, nine of them evolved from a "rough" to a "precise" status, with only one showing no change.

The 10 mutation was in eight antigens; these antigens were aligned, and the result was shown in **Figure 5**.

Let us ask why the detection limit for the wild type D614 SARS-CoV-2 was 21.5 copies; for Omicron, it was 14.3 copies, but for the Delta subtype, it raised to 32.0 copies [8].

The Delta subtype is the most difficult to detect, and this is to say the virus is most difficult to stay in the upper respiratory tract; instead, it is easy to deep in the lungs. The virus must have a loading amount to reach the detection limit. The increased loading virus caused more virulence. Most of the patients need oxygen. The need required oxygen was so huge that the news was reported about it in India in October 2020.

The possible reason for the increased virulence might be due to the Antibody Enhanced Effects (ADE). The previously generated low precession antibody will help the high precession antigen of Delta subtype enter the human body and cause inflammation.

At least 92.31% of the whole antigens had evolved from "rough" to "precise", and only 7.69% showed no change. The whole antigen mutation in the Delta subtype determined the virulence of the virus.

4.3.2 The whole mutation antigens in Omicron subtype were at least 30 site mutations

The limit of the detection for the wild type D614 SARS-CoV-2 was 21.5 copies; for Omicron, it was 14.3 copies, but for the Delta subtype, it raised to 32.0 copies [8].

Omicron is easy to detect; this is to say the virus is easy to stay in the mouth but not easily deep in the lungs. Less virus loading will be found in the assays to reach the detection limit. And the less-loading virus caused weak virulence. The virulence should be weak in the Omicron strain. The virulence of Omicron was so weak, that many patients did not need any treatment.

Whole mutations antigen fragment in Omicron was over 30, but for most of them, the antigen precessions were decreased. If the majority of precessions were decreased, the whole precession would be displayed decreased, and the virulence of the virus would also decrease.

The previous high precession antibody will avoid the ADE when it meets the low antigen in the Omicron subtype.

The whole antigen mutation in the Omicron subtype determined the virulence of the virus.

4.3.3 Zero mutated antigen in D614 original wild subtype

The distribution rate of wild type in the up respiratory tract should be between Delta and Omicron. The distribution rate in the lung should also be between Delta type and Omicron type. The loading virus could be between the two. The virulence should be between those two types also.

Zero mutated D614 wild strain should have the basic virulence.

4.3.4 Whole mutated antigen in D614G subtype

This whole mutation was the same as the longest fragment mutation because it had only one mutation. The infectivity, for sure, was increased. There was a report that the D614G patients had a higher rate of entering the intensive care unit (ICU) than D614 patients [2].

To sum up, just like D614 mutated to D614G, the Delta subtype of SARS-CoV-2 started to conduct its evolution in "rough" status fragments. The final goal for evolution was the "precise" status.

The mutations in the Omicron types of SARS-CoV-2 also follow such rules, and we would like to discuss this in other papers.

According to our hypothesis, the "common precise" with high precession antigens of the SARS-CoV-2 could be designed in silicon, developed in a laboratory, and confirmed in animal models.

Such "common precise" antigens could be used to develop "common precise" antibodies. If the "common precise" antibodies were used in the antigen test, all the various antigens with lower or the same precise degrees could be detected. One antibody could detect numerous lower precession antigens, even the antigens not mutated yet now, but will be mutated in the next 3 years.

The evolution of antigens from "rough" status to "precise", has two meanings. The first meaning is that, like a trip, the departure site starts first from the most "rough" antigen and last from the most "precise" antigen. The longest fragments did this work to determine virus infectivity. The second meaning is that the "rough" antigen's evolution destination to "precise" antigens. The whole mutation antigens did this work to determine the virulence. This paper did focus on both topics. Beside for forecast mutation, understanding such rules of evolution can also help the development of reagents for detecting both "rough" and "precise" antigens, or even help with the development of the vaccines against SARS-CoV-2, as well as other infectious diseases. And finally, this information could help to control of the Covid-19, other epidemic infectious diseases, and tumors.

5. Conclusion

The longest antigen fragments determined virus infectivity. Whole mutated fragments determined the virulence. Both were associated with different mutated fragments with varied antigen precession in the Delta subtype of SARS-CoV-2.

Acknowledgements

This work was supported by project NTF21021, Research Starting Funding from Shantou University, and project 220513116490768, Medical Health Issue in Technical Plan from Shantou Science Technical Bureau.

Author contributions

Peijun Zuo searched for the information, performed the analysis, and wrote the paper. Professor Dr. Liping Li provided the key advice. Longlong Zuo and Zhihong Li did an interpretation of the data.

Conflicts of interest

The authors declare no conflicts of interest.

Research ethics approval

This is not a traditional epidemiological study to find the relation between protein molecules and the epidemic disease caused by the protein mutation. It did not contain any samples from humans and animals. A research ethics approval is not applicable.

Abbreviations

A	alanine
C	cysteine
COVID-19	coronavirus disease 2019
D	aspartate
E	glutamate
F	phenylalanine
G	glycine
H	histidine
I	isoleucine
K	lysine
L	leucine

M	methionine
N	asparagine
P	proline
Q	glutamine
R	arginine
S	serine
SARS-CoV-2	Severe Acute Respiratory Syndrome Corona Virus 2
SD	standard deviation
T	threonine
W	tryptophan
V	valine
Y	tyrosine

Key points

Question: Were the virulence and infectivity associated with different fragments in the Delta subtype of SARS-CoV-2? **Findings:** The longest antigen fragments determined virus infectivity. Whole mutated fragments determined the virulence mutated from "rough" status to "precise", with only one in ten showing no change. **Meaning:** In a SARS-CoV-2 pandemic, the SD of the molecular weight of amino acids, the indicator of "precession", may be used to forecast the coming mutations. The longest D614 fragment, N148 fragment, and I358 fragment determined the infectivity. The whole mutations determined the virulence.

Author details

Peijun Zuo[1*], Longlong Zuo[2], Zhihong Li[1] and Liping Li[1*]

1 Shantou University, Guangdong, China

2 The Chinese University of Hong Kong, Hong Kong, China

*Address all correspondence to: peijunzuo@hotmail.com and lpli@stu.edu.cn

References

[1] Zhou P et al. A pneumonia outbreak associated with a new coronavirus of probable bat origin. Nature. 2020; **579**(7798):270-273

[2] Korber B et al. Tracking changes in SARS-CoV-2 spike: Evidence that D614G increases infectivity of the COVID-19 virus. Cell. 2020;**182**(4):812-827 e19

[3] Jhun H et al. SARS-CoV-2 Delta (B.1.617.2) variant: A unique T478K mutation in receptor binding motif (RBM) of spike gene. Immune Network. 2021;**21**(5):e32

[4] Yadav PD et al. Neutralization of variant under investigation B.1.617.1 with sera of BBV152 Vaccinees. Clinical Infectious Diseases. 2022;**74**(2): 366-368

[5] Pascarella S et al. SARS-CoV-2 B.1.617 Indian variants: Are electrostatic potential changes responsible for a higher transmission rate? Journal of Medical Virology. 2021;**93**(12):6551-6556

[6] Planas D et al. Reduced sensitivity of SARS-CoV-2 variant Delta to antibody neutralization. Nature. 2021;**596**(7871): 276-280

[7] Wu J et al. The antigenicity of SARS-CoV-2 Delta variants aggregated 10 high-frequency mutations in RBD has not changed sufficiently to replace the current vaccine strain. Signal Transduction and Targeted Therapy. 2022;7(1):18

[8] Tsui WNT et al. Molecular detection of SARS-CoV-2 and differentiation of omicron and Delta variant strains. Transboundary and Emerging Diseases. Sep 2022;**69**(5):e1618-e1631. DOI: 10.1111/tbed.14497. Epub 2022 Mar 13. PMID: 35218683; PMCID: PMC9115370

[9] Mazhar MW et al. Detection of SARS-CoV-2 by using real-time PCR nasopharyngeal swabs in suspected patients and their clinical medication. Sensors International. 2022;**3**:100148

[10] Kannan SR et al. Evolutionary analysis of the Delta and Delta Plus variants of the SARS-CoV-2 viruses. Journal of Autoimmunity. 2021;**124**: 102715

[11] Nunes DR et al. Deep phylogenetic-based clustering analysis uncovers new and shared mutations in SARS-CoV-2 variants as a result of directional and convergent evolution. PLoS One. 2022; **17**(5):e0268389

[12] Hirabara SM et al. SARS-COV-2 variants: Differences and potential of immune evasion. Frontiers in Cellular and Infection Microbiology. 2021;**11**: 781429

[13] Yao H et al. Molecular architecture of the SARS-CoV-2 virus. Cell. 2020; **183**(3):730-738 e13

[14] Zuo P, Zuo L, Li Z et al. Antigen evolution from D614, to G614, to Delta, and to Omicron subtype of SARS-CoV-2. 03 August 2022. DOI: 10.21203/rs.3.rs-1859710/v1. PREPRINT (Version 1) available at Research Square

[15] Meng Q et al. Spiralin-like protein SLP31 from Spiroplasma eriocheiris as a potential antigen for immunodiagnostics of tremor disease in Chinese mitten crab Eriocheir sinensis. Folia Microbiologia (Praha). 2010;**55**(3):245-250

Chapter 6

Unraveling the Significance of Phage-Derived Enzymes for Treating Secondary Bacterial Infections among COVID-19 Patients

Amina Nazir, Lulu Li, Xiaonan Zhao, Yuqing Liu and Yibao Chen

Abstract

The COVID-19 (Corona Virus Disease of 2019) pandemic had a profound impact on humanity, affecting over 200 million people. Among the complications associated with viral respiratory infections in COVID-19 patients, secondary bacterial infections (SBIs) pose a significant threat to the prognosis of COVID-19 patients, leading to increased morbidity and mortality rates. This crisis is exacerbated by the growing antimicrobial resistance in bacteria, which limits our available treatment options. Recently, the use of phage and phage-derived enzymes (PDEs) has emerged as a promising alternative strategy to combat bacterial infections as they possess a natural ability to eliminate bacteria effectively. The primary objective of this chapter is to emphasize the prevalence of SBIs and the significance of PDEs in addressing SBIs among COVID-19 patients. Specifically, phage-derived depolymerases and endolysins showed considerable antivirulence potency and effectively break down the bacterial cell wall. These enzymes have emerged as a promising class of new antibiotics, with their therapeutic efficacy already confirmed in animal models. By exploring this novel approach, we may discover new avenues to improve patient outcomes and combat the challenges posed by bacterial infections in the context of the COVID-19 pandemic.

Keywords: bacterial infection, phage enzymes, COVID-19 pathogenic, secondary bacterial infections, patients

1. Introduction

The COVID-19 (Corona Virus Disease of 2019) pandemic has had a profound impact on global health, overwhelming healthcare systems and resulting in significant morbidity and mortality rates worldwide [1]. While the primary focus has been on managing the viral infection caused by severe acute respiratory syndrome coronavirus 2 (SARS-CoV-2), it has become increasingly evident that secondary bacterial infections (SBIs) pose an additional challenge in the clinical management of COVID-19 patients [2]. Compared to pneumonia caused by other respiratory pathogens, severe COVID-19, resulting from infection with the severe acute respiratory syndrome SARS-CoV-2, is known to be associated with a prolonged duration of illness and causes SBIs [3]. These secondary infections can complicate the course of the disease, prolong hospital stays, and contribute to adverse patient outcomes. Patients who experience extended hospital stays face an elevated risk of acquiring multidrug-resistant (MDR) bacterial infections within healthcare settings [4]. These infections are often a result of nosocomial transmission and inadequate antibiotic treatment. Furthermore, the widespread and intensive use of antibiotics during the pandemic can contribute to a higher prevalence of MDR bacteria [5]. Conventional antibiotics have been the cornerstone of bacterial infection treatment for decades, but their efficacy is diminishing due to the emergence of antibiotic-resistant bacteria. The urgent need for novel therapeutic approaches has prompted researchers to explore alternative strategies [6]. One such approach gaining traction is the use of phage-derived enzymes (PDEs) as potential tools to combat bacterial infections.

Phage therapy, which utilizes bacteriophages (phages) as natural predators of bacteria, has emerged as a promising avenue for the treatment of bacterial infections [7, 8]. Phages are viruses that specifically target and infect bacteria, ultimately leading to their destruction [9–11]. Phages have the ability to recognize and attach to bacterial cell surfaces, inject their genetic material into the bacteria, and hijack the host machinery to produce numerous progeny phages. As a result, phage therapy has shown efficacy against a wide range of bacterial pathogens [12]. Phage therapy and PDEs have not been documented in previous viral pandemics. Currently, there are few efforts have been done on the application of phage therapy in COVID-19 patients with secondary carbapenem-resistant *Acinetobacter baumannii* (CRAB) pneumonia [13]. Adaptive Phage Therapeutics, a clinical-stage biotechnology company, has recently initiated a study to explore the use of phages in treating COVID-19 patients with bacterial co-infections [14]. However, there are also few drawbacks and limitations of using phages as alternatives [15].

In the context of COVID-19, the significance of PDEs (endolysins and depolymerases) in managing SBIs is of particular interest [16]. As COVID-19 patients often experience compromised immune responses and respiratory distress, they are susceptible to SBIs, which can lead to severe complications and worsen patient outcomes [3]. Therefore, understanding the potential role of PDEs in mitigating these secondary infections is crucial for improving therapeutic interventions and patient care. These enzymes have specific mechanisms of action that allow them to target and eliminate bacteria in a highly efficient manner [17–20].

This chapter aims to unravel the significance of PDEs in SBIs among COVID-19 patients. We will try to shed light on the occurrence of SBIs in COVID-19, factors that can enhance the susceptibility to SBIs. We will provide insights into the advantages and limitations of utilizing PDEs for controlling such infections and a practical work flow for working with PDEs as well. By shedding light on this topic, this chapter seeks to contribute to the growing body of knowledge surrounding the use of PDEs as a novel therapeutic strategy against SBIs in the context of COVID-19.

2. Fundamental concerns about high prevalence of SBIs in COVID-19 patients

COVID-19 has emerged as a potentially life-threatening infectious disease, prompting scientists to intensify their efforts in comprehending its pathogenesis [21]. The significant morbidity and mortality rates associated with COVID-19 primarily stem from the widespread presence of the SARS-CoV-2 and subsequent microbial infections within the respiratory system [22]. The higher rates of SBIs in COVID-19 patients have emerged as a primary concern in the medical community. The correlation between contracting COVID-19 and developing subsequent bacterial infections has already been confirmed. There is a rising trend of simultaneous severe bacterial infections alongside the viral disease in COVID-19 patients, leading to prolonged hospital stays [23]. This scenario can potentially exacerbate the severity of COVID-19 illness and contribute to high mortality rates [24].

The most commonly encountered pathogens causing SBIs in COVID-19 patients include *Acinetobacter baumannii (A. baumannii), Pseudomonas aeruginosa (P. aeruginosa), Klebsiella pneumoniae (K. pneumoniae), and Staphylococcus aureus (S. aureus)*. The isolation ratios of carbapenem-resistant and colistin-resistant strains for these pathogens are as follows: *A. baumannii*: 83.7% of isolates were carbapenem-resistant and 5.6% were colistin-resistant. For *P. aeruginosa*: 79.2% of isolates were carbapenem-resistant and 1.7% were colistin-resistant and *K. pneumoniae*: 42.7% of isolates were carbapenem-resistant and 42.7% were colistin-resistant [25]. While some COVID-19 patients experienced a higher incidence of bloodstream infections (BSI) caused by *Enterococcus*, this was not a general trend. Whole-genome sequencing of *Enterococcus* isolates revealed that the increased rate of BSI in these patients could not be solely attributed to nosocomial transmission [26].

In a multicenter study involving 476 COVID-19 participants, the results demonstrated that SBIs were strongly associated with the severity of outcomes [2]. Based on evidence from previous pandemics and seasonal flu outbreaks, it has been suggested that co-infections have the potential to exacerbate viral illnesses. However, it remains unclear whether they definitively impact patient outcomes in the case of COVID-19. During the initial SARS-CoV outbreak in 2003, up to 30% of patients were found to have SBIs, and co-infection was positively associated with disease severity [27]. Another study revealed that bacterial co-infections were found in 2–65% of patients during regular influenza seasons, and these co-infections were associated with elevated levels of illness and mortality [28]. The escalation of bacterial co-infections during seasonal flu emphasizes the importance of investigating the underlying mechanisms of pathogenicity, particularly in the context of COVID-19.

In a retrospective study conducted by Zhou et al., it was reported that during the ongoing COVID-19 pandemic, approximately one in seven hospitalized patients with the illness experienced a potentially life-threatening SBIs. Among the non-survivors, almost half of them (27 out of 54) developed a secondary infection. Additionally, 10 out of 32 patients (31%) developed ventilator-associated pneumonia, which required invasive mechanical ventilation [29]. These findings highlight the significant risk of SBIs in COVID-19 patients, particularly in those who require intensive care and mechanical ventilation. Several studies have indicated that COVID-19 patients experience more severe illness and a higher fatality rate compared to patients with influenza [30]. In fact, the fatality rate among COVID-19 patients has been reported to be approximately three times higher than that of influenza patients [31]. Furthermore, COVID-19 patients exhibited a two-fold increase in patient mortality rates associated with pulmonary SBIs. In comparison to influenza infections, COVID-19 patients require a longer duration from admission to the detection of bacterial growth. These observations highlight the heightened risk and impact of SBIs in the context of COVID-19, underscoring the need for effective management strategies to mitigate their consequences. Based on a meta-analysis of 24 cohort studies involving 3338 hospitalized COVID-19 patients, it was found that 3.5% of patients (with 95% confidence interval (CI) ranging from 0.4% to 6.7%) had bacterial co-infection at the time of presentation. Additionally, 14.3% of patients (with 95% CI ranging from 9.6% to 18.9%) developed SBIs [32]. These findings provide an estimation of the prevalence of bacterial co-infections and SBIs in hospitalized COVID-19 patients, highlighting the need for vigilance in managing these additional complications. According to the results of microbial culture tests, a total of 92 patients (8.7%) had microbiologically confirmed respiratory or circulatory tract infections. Among 61 patients evaluated for respiratory tract infections, 44 patients were identified to have mono-microbial infections, while 17 patients had poly-microbial infections [33]. These findings indicate the presence of both single and multiple bacterial pathogens contributing to respiratory tract infections in a subset of patients. Out of the 94 patients included in the study, a substantial majority, approximately 68%, acquired at least one of the studied SBIs during their stay in the intensive care unit (ICU). Among these patients, nearly two-thirds (65.96%, n = 62) developed secondary pneumonia as a specific type of SBI [34].

COVID-19 patients exhibited higher rates of bacterial infections compared to other pneumonia patients, with rates of 12.6% versus 8.7%, respectively. The duration of bacterial infection was also longer in COVID-19 patients, with a median of 4 (range 1–8) days compared to 1 (range 1–3) day in other pneumonia patients. Notably, Gram-positive infections that developed later (more than 48 hours after admission) were more frequent in COVID-19 patients, accounting for 28% compared to 9.5% in other pneumonia patients [35]. Importantly, for COVID-19 patients, the presence of SBIs was associated with a 2.7-fold increased risk of death. This highlights the significant impact of secondary infections on the prognosis and mortality of COVID-19 patients. According to Zhang et al., their study revealed that 22 out of 38 patients (57.89%) experienced secondary infections. The likelihood of developing secondary infections was higher in patients who underwent invasive mechanical ventilation or were in critical condition ($P < 0.0001$) [36]. The presence of secondary infections was associated with lower rates of discharge and increased mortality rates. These findings suggest that secondary infections in COVID-19 patients can have a negative impact on patient outcomes, leading to prolonged hospital stays, increased mortality, and potentially hampering the recovery process.

Based on several disease severity markers, it has been observed that COVID-19 patients tend to experience more severe illnesses and have worse outcomes. This is evident from a higher percentage of patients requiring intubation for mechanical ventilation and an increased number of deaths [37]. These markers suggest a greater impact and high severity of COVID-19 compared to other respiratory illnesses. Significantly, COVID-19 patients have been found to have a higher incidence of SBIs than previously described, and these infections have been independently associated with death in COVID-19 cases [5]. These findings suggest that SBIs may play a significant role in the severity of the disease in COVID-19 patients and could even be a potential target for therapeutic interventions.

3. Major factors that can enhance the susceptibility to SBIs in COVID-19 patients

SBIs can cause severe complications in patients with COVID-19 as follows:

3.1 Prolonged hospitalization and invasive procedures

Many severe cases of COVID-19 require hospitalization, often ICUs. Prolonged hospital stays and invasive procedures, such as intubation and mechanical ventilation, central venous catheter insertion, or urinary catheterization, increase the risk of nosocomial (hospital-acquired) bacterial infections [38]. These procedures can introduce bacteria into the body or provide opportunities for bacterial colonization. Additionally, COVID-19 patients who receive immunosuppressive treatments, such as tocilizumab, anakinra, and corticosteroids, have been found to have a higher incidence of BSIs [16]. This has led to increased mortality rates and a greater need for ICU admissions among patients with BSI. Moreover, COVID-19 infection triggers pathological alterations in the body, such as a compromised immune system, dysregulated immune signaling, and diffuse alveolar damage [26]. These factors contribute to the development of SBIs and limit the effectiveness of antibiotic treatments. The combination of COVID-19 induced immune dysfunction and SBIs poses significant challenges in the management of critically ill patients, requiring a multifaceted approach to optimize outcomes.

3.2 Antimicrobial resistance (AMR)

The convergence of AMR crises poses significant threats when dealing with SBIs in COVID-19-affected patients. Antimicrobial usage is crucial in the treatment of infectious diseases. However, the indiscriminate use of antibiotics during the COVID-19 outbreak has exacerbated the problem of AMR. Despite the widespread administration of antibiotic therapy, the increased prevalence of SBIs in COVID-19 patients may be attributed to the presence of AMR bacteria in hospital settings [39]. The most frequently identified infections in blood and mucous samples of COVID-19 patients are associated with *ESKAPE* pathogens, which include *Enterococcus faecium, S. aureus, K. pneumoniae, A. baumannii, P. aeruginosa*, and *Enterobacter* species. In the context of influenza illness, *S. aureus* pathogens have been known to cause secondary pneumonia. Environmental changes and immunological responses that create favorable conditions for *S. aureus* infection are considered factors contributing to its spread to the lungs. Additionally, *A. baumannii* has been associated with long-term respiratory conditions predisposing individuals to influenza-like upper respiratory tract infections [40]. *P. aeruginosa* is frequently encountered as an opportunistic pathogen in the respiratory system. Nevertheless, it is also acknowledged as the predominant Gram-negative bacterial specie linked to severe hospital-acquired infections in diverse healthcare environments [41]. Its ability to cause infections in hospital environments poses a significant concern due to its inherent resistance to many antibiotics and its propensity for developing resistance mechanisms. Effective control measures and judicious use of antibiotics are essential in mitigating the impact of *P. aeruginosa* infections in healthcare settings. ICUs and patients with compromised immune systems are particularly susceptible to nosocomial infections caused by Gram-negative bacteria such as *A. baumannii* and *K. pneumoniae*, both of which exhibit signs of MDR. Among the microorganisms isolated from blood cultures, coagulase-negative *staphylococci* accounted for 31% of cases, while *A. baumannii* was prominent at 27.5%. In respiratory tract cultures, *A. baumannii* constituted the majority with a rate of 33.3%, followed by *S. aureus* and *K. pneumoniae*, each at 9.5%. Notably, *A. baumannii* exhibited the highest level of resistance, being resistant to all antibiotics except for colistin [33]. This highlights the challenging nature of treating infections caused by MDR *A. baumannii* and the importance of appropriate infection control measures to prevent their spread in healthcare settings. Indeed, the availability of effective antibiotic options for "superbugs" such as MDR bacteria is limited [16]. Compounding the issue, the use of certain "last-resort" antibiotics, including colistin, is closely regulated due to concerns regarding organ toxicity, disruption of normal microbial flora, and the potential for inducing AMR [42]. This creates a challenging situation in managing infections caused by these highly resistant bacteria, as alternative treatment options are often limited and their use must be carefully considered to minimize adverse effects. This highlights the urgent need for the development of new antimicrobial therapies and the implementation of strategies to combat the spread of AMR.

3.3 Impaired immune response

COVID-19 can suppress the immune system, making individuals more susceptible to SBIs. The viral infection and the resulting inflammatory response can disrupt the normal functioning of immune cells, impairing their ability to fight off bacterial pathogens effectively [43, 44].

3.4 Ventilator-associated pneumonia (VAP)

COVID-19 patients who require mechanical ventilation are at higher risk of developing VAP [45, 46]. VAP caused by bacteria that colonize the respiratory tract and can lead to serious lung infections. The use of ventilators can impair normal lung function and create an environment conducive to bacterial growth, increasing the likelihood of VAP.

3.5 Disruption of the normal microbiota

COVID-19 and its treatments, such as broad-spectrum antibiotics, can disrupt the normal balance of microbial communities in the body [47, 48]. This disruption, known as dysbiosis, can create opportunities for pathogenic bacteria to overgrow and cause infections.

3.6 Pre-existing comorbidities

COVID-19 patients often have pre-existing health conditions, such as diabetes, cardiovascular diseases, or chronic respiratory conditions. These comorbidities can weaken the immune system and impair the body's ability to combat bacterial infections effectively [49, 50].

3.7 Viral-induced tissue damage

The SARS-CoV-2 virus primarily infects the respiratory tract, causing inflammation and damage to lung tissues. This tissue damage can compromise the local defense mechanisms and create an environment favorable for bacterial colonization and infection [51]. Healthcare professionals take precautions to minimize the risk of SBIs in COVID-19 patients, including appropriate antibiotic use, infection control measures, and monitoring for signs of infection.

4. Harnessing the potential of PDEs as alternative therapeutics

Considering the sluggish pace of new antibiotic discovery, intact phages and their proteins emerge as promising therapeutic options for antibiotic-resistant bacteria [52–54]. The concept of phage therapy dates back to the early twentieth century, but it has regained interest in recent years due to the rise of AMR. Phage therapy, utilizing phages, has gained attention as a potential alternative to conventional antibiotics [55]. Phages have several advantages over traditional antibiotics, including their specificity to target bacteria, ability to self-replicate, and potential to evolve alongside bacteria. Clinical trials and case studies have demonstrated the efficacy of phage therapy in treating various bacterial infections, including those caused by MDR bacteria [56]. However, there are some potential drawbacks and challenges associated with their use including AMR transfer, emergence of phage-resistant bacteria, immunogenicity and safety concerns, complex biology, and regulatory challenges. In this context, there has been considerable research focused on phage-encoded proteins that show potential in combating bacterial infections. They have shown efficacy against a wide range of bacterial pathogens, including both Gram-positive and Gram-negative bacteria. These enzymes exhibit a high degree of specificity and can rapidly kill bacteria without harming host cells or disrupting the normal microbiota. These PDEs included endolysins and depolymerases, use as potential therapeutic agents [57]. Endolysins are enzymes produced by phages during the lytic cycle. They can hydrolyze the bacterial cell wall, leading to bacterial lysis and death [58]. Depolymerases are enzymes that degrade the extracellular polymeric substances in biofilms, which are protective matrices formed by bacteria (**Figure 1**) [59].

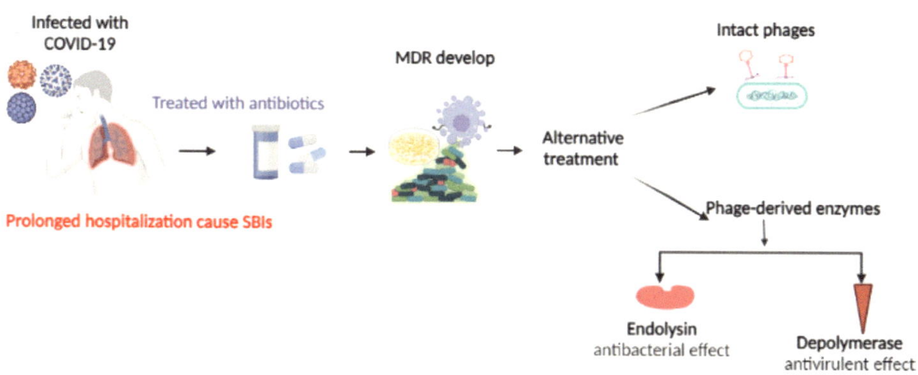

Figure 1.
A schematic representation of drug-resistant secondary infections that can occur in patients infected with severe acute respiratory syndrome coronavirus 2 (SARS-CoV-2).

Studies have shown that PDEs can effectively eradicate bacterial biofilms, making them potential candidates for treating biofilm-related infections [60]. They have demonstrated activity against antibiotic-resistant bacteria, including methicillin-resistant *S. aureus* and carbapenem-resistant *Enterobacteriaceae* [61]. In addition to their direct antimicrobial effects, PDEs can synergize with antibiotics, enhancing their efficacy against bacterial pathogens [62]. These enzymes have shown promising in various applications, including wound healing, food safety, agriculture, and the prevention of bacterial contamination in medical devices [63]. PDEs are generally considered safe, with a low risk of adverse effects. However, more research is needed to fully understand their long-term safety profiles.

However, challenges regarding development and applications of PDEs include regulatory hurdles, formulation optimization, and the potential for bacterial resistance to emerge [64]. Strategies such as engineering enzymes for improved stability and activity, as well as combination therapies with antibiotics or other antimicrobial agents, may help overcome these challenges.

5. PDEs to act as anti-virulence agents: depolymerases & endolysins

PDEs, such as endolysins and depolymerases, possess a unique mechanisms of action to target and eliminate bacterial pathogens (**Figure 2**). These enzymes have evolved to efficiently disrupt bacterial cell walls or biofilm matrices, ultimately leading to bacterial death.

5.1 Endolysins

Endolysins are bacteriophage-encoded enzymes that target the peptidoglycan layer of bacterial cell walls. They have a modular structure, typically consisting of two functional domains: an N-terminal catalytic domain and a C-terminal cell

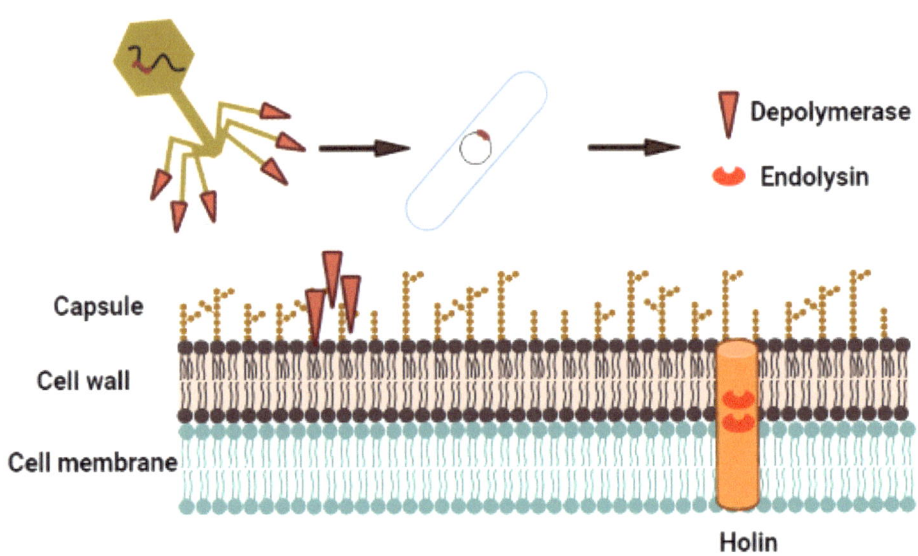

Figure 2.
Mechanism of action of phage-derived enzymes (PDEs).

wall-binding domain. The catalytic domain possesses enzymatic activity, such as amidase or glycosidase activity, which can cleave specific bonds within the peptidoglycan structure. Once the endolysin binds to the cell wall of susceptible bacteria, the catalytic domain hydrolyzes the peptidoglycan, leading to the rapid breakdown of the cell wall. The loss of structural integrity causes the bacteria to lyse, releasing progeny phages into the surrounding environment [65].

5.2 Depolymerases

Depolymerases are enzymes produced by phages that target the EPS of bacterial biofilms. Biofilms are complex communities of bacteria encased in a self-produced matrix of EPS, which protects them from the immune system and antimicrobial agents. Depolymerases specifically degrade the EPS components, disrupting the biofilm matrix and rendering bacteria more susceptible to clearance by the immune system or antimicrobial treatments. Depending on the specific type of biofilm and bacterial species, depolymerases can degrade various components of the EPS, such as polysaccharides, proteins, or DNA. Capsular depolymerases present a unique form of antibiotic action: rather than killing bacteria outright, they strip the bacteria of their protective polysaccharides, rendering them vulnerable to immune factors. This characteristic provides a potential edge over endolysins, as depolymerases do not cause bacterial lysis, thereby reducing the risk of inflammatory responses caused by endotoxins [66].

To date, there is limited research about in vivo studies of PDEs, but their efficacy has been demonstrated in animal models (**Table 1**). The results indicate that PDEs have the potential to revolutionize the treatment of secondary infections in COVID-19 patients who are unresponsive to conventional therapies.

Phage	Enzyme	Delivery route	Model	Results	Reference
S. aureus phage SAP-26	LysSAP26	5–80 μg/mL injection	Mouse model	40% survival rate	[67]
S. aureus phage	SAL200	Intranasal	Lethal murine model	40% survival rate	[68]
E. coli K1	Endo Sialidase from Coliphage E	Intraperitoneal injection	Neonatal rat model of bacteremia	100% of animals protected from death	[69]
Salmonella Typhimurium	P22sTsp endorhamnosidase from *Salmonella* phage P22	Oral administration	Chicken model of gastrointestinal infection	Bacterial cfu reduction of ~1 order	[70]
A. baumannii phage PD-6A3	Ply6A3	Intraperitoneal injection	Mouse sepsis model	32.4% killed	[71]
K. pneumoniae	K64dep capsule depolymerase from *Klebsiella* phage K64-1	Intraperitoneal injection	Mouse model of bacteremia	100% of animals protected from death	[72]

Phage	Enzyme	Delivery route	Model	Results	Reference
A. baumannii phage vB_AbaP_D2	Abtn-4	Intraperitoneal injection	Mouse sepsis model	*A. baumannii* were killed by Abtn-4 (5 μM) in 2 h	[73]
P. aeruginosa	LKA1gp49 LPS lyase from *Pseudomonas* phage LKA1	Injection into the last pro-leg	*Galleria mellonella* infection model	20% of animals protected from death	[15]
K. pneumoniae	Dep_kpv79 and Dep_kpv767 depolymerase	Intraperitoneal injection, intramuscular injection	Mouse model	80%, 100%	[74]
A. baumannii	depolymerase Dpo71	Injection into the last pro-leg	*Galleria mellonella* infection model	80%	[75]
A. baumannii	Capsule depolymerase B9gp69	—	Cell line model of human lung	—	[76]
Proteus mirabilis	Phage derived-Depolymerase	Injection into the last pro-leg	*Galleria mellonella* infection model	20% protected from death	[77]
ESKAPE *group bacteria*	LysAm24, LysAp22, LysECD7, and LysSi3	Injection	Mouse model	40% of animals	[78]

Table 1.
Applications of phage-derived enzymes in animal models.

6. A practical approach for PDEs regarding COVID-19

To effectively implement phage-derived therapeutics in a COVID-19-designated hospital, a practical workflow involving different functional areas and varying levels of personal protective equipment (PPE) can be established. The following steps outline a feasible workflow.

6.1 Patient care and bacterial culture

Standard patient care and bacterial culture activities will predominantly occur in the patient ward and clinical laboratory, utilizing appropriate PPE for infection control.

6.2 Phage screening and efficiency analysis

Within the clinical laboratory, a dedicated section adhering to BSL-3 lab PPE requirements will be designated for conducting phage screening and efficiency analysis. This specialized area ensures safety during phage-related procedures.

DOI: http://dx.doi.org/10.5772/intechopen.1002618

6.3 Phage amplification and vial preparation

Phages will be regularly amplified by cultivating them in the original host bacteria within the standard microbiology laboratory. This process, carried out under appropriate PPE, will result in the production of ready-to-use phage vials.

6.4 Packaging facility

A packaging facility, meeting Good Manufacturing Practice (GMP) certification standards, will be responsible for packaging the phage vials. This controlled environment ensures quality and safety during the packaging process.

6.5 Selection and delivery of therapeutic proteins

Qualified vials containing purified PDEs will be efficiently selected from the packaging facility. These selected vials will be promptly delivered to the patient ward for therapeutic administration. This process follows a controlled material flow, moving from lower BSL lab zones to higher BSL lab zones, accompanied by the necessary information flow.

6.6 Phage-typing and epidemiological analysis

Bacterial isolates will undergo regular phage-typing procedures for epidemiological purposes. This analysis will provide valuable data to inform the development of sufficient quantities of PDEs and the creation of broad-spectrum, fixed-composition cocktails, particularly for emergency situations. By implementing this practicable workflow, a COVID-19-designated hospital can effectively integrate phage-derived therapeutics into its existing healthcare infrastructure, ensuring safety, quality, and expedited delivery of these potential treatments to patients in need (**Figure 3**).

7. Challenges and future prospects

Although PDEs show promise as a therapeutic strategy, several challenges need to be addressed. This section discusses the limitations and obstacles associated with their utilization, including regulatory hurdles, bacterial resistance, and formulation issues. Furthermore, it explores potential future directions and advancements in the field.

7.1 Regulatory hurdles

One of the key challenges in the clinical implementation of PDEs is navigating the regulatory landscape. Regulatory agencies may have limited experience or specific requirements for the approval and use of phage-based therapies, which can impede their widespread adoption. Overcoming these regulatory hurdles requires collaborative efforts between researchers, regulatory bodies, and pharmaceutical companies to establish clear guidelines and streamline the approval process [64, 79].

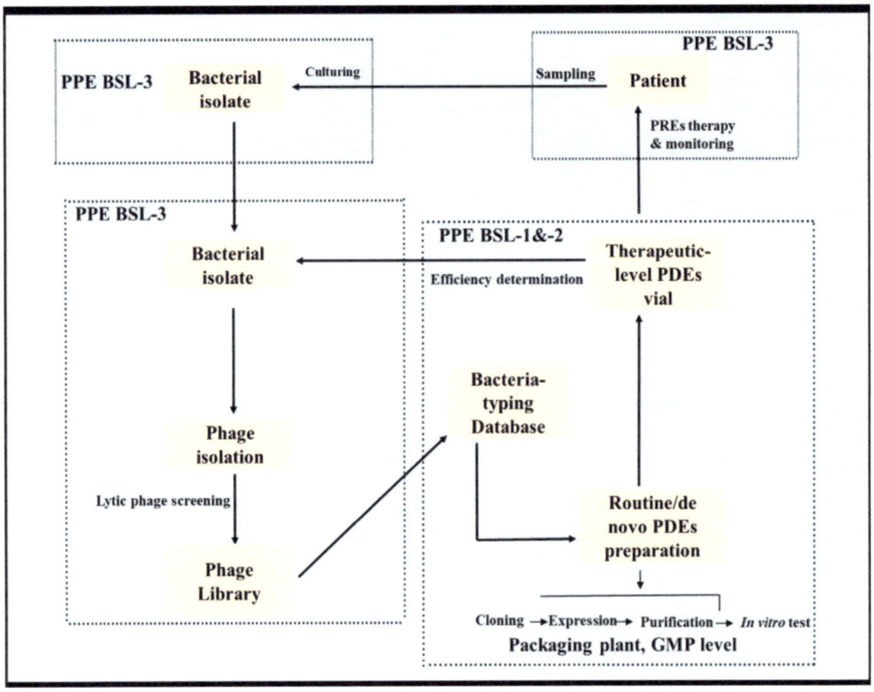

Figure 3.
This study proposes a workflow for managing COVID-19 (Corona virus disease of 2019) infections [16]. It involves using a pre-established phage library targeted against a specific pathogenic bacterium that has been identified in either a patient or on a hospital surface. The process includes screening the phage library and delivering pre-stocked phage-enzyme vials for application to the patient or the affected environment. PDEs: phage-derived enzyme; PPE: personal protective equipment; BSL: biosafety level; and GMP: good manufacturing practices.

7.2 Bacterial resistance

As with any antimicrobial treatment, the potential emergence of bacterial resistance to PDEs is a concern. Bacteria can evolve mechanisms to evade the activity of these enzymes, such as modifying their cell surface receptors or producing protective substances. Continued research is needed to understand the mechanisms of bacterial resistance to PDEs and develop strategies to mitigate its occurrence, such as using multiple enzymes or combinations with other antimicrobials [56].

7.3 Formulation and delivery optimization

Effective delivery of PDEs to the target site remains a challenge. Enzymes must be formulated in a way that maintains their stability, activity, and bioavailability. Overcoming barriers such as enzymatic degradation, poor penetration into tissues, and immunogenicity requires innovative delivery systems, including nanoparticles, liposomes, or hydrogels, to ensure optimal enzyme delivery and efficacy [80, 81].

7.4 Clinical trials and evidentiary support

Additional clinical trials are necessary to establish the safety, effectiveness, and ideal dosing protocols of PDEs in treating SBIs among patients with COVID-19.

Robust clinical evidence is necessary to demonstrate their effectiveness compared to standard treatments, including antibiotics. Well-designed clinical trials with appropriate control groups and endpoints are crucial for gathering the data required to support the integration of PDEs into clinical practice.

7.5 Personalized and precision medicine

The development of personalized treatment approaches, guided by patient-specific bacterial profiles and susceptibilities, holds promise for optimizing the use of PDEs. Integrating genomics and metagenomics techniques to characterize bacterial populations and predict their response to specific enzymes could enable tailored treatment strategies. Implementing precision medicine principles can help optimize therapy, minimize the emergence of resistance, and improve patient outcomes.

Overall, despite the challenges, the future prospects of PDEs in SBIs among COVID-19 patients are promising. Addressing the regulatory hurdles, understanding and countering bacterial resistance, and delivery systems, generating robust clinical evidence, exploring combination therapy strategies, and embracing personalized medicine approaches will contribute to realizing the full potential of PDEs as valuable therapeutic tools in the management of SBIs in the context of COVID-19 and beyond.

8. Conclusion

The end of the COVID-19 pandemic is expected to be a prolonged process, despite extensive efforts made to control it. Various indicators of disease severity have revealed that certain COVID-19 patients experience more severe illness and worse outcomes. Additionally, our ability to combat MDR bacteria is diminishing as they become more widespread, further exacerbating the complications in COVID-19 patients. Although there have been limited clinical studies on SBIs in COVID-19, the findings suggest that the condition might be treatable. To address challenges like resistance, host specificity, and drug development during the purification and characterization of phage-derived antimicrobials, alternative phage-based treatments can be utilized when the complete phage is not as effective. The significance of PDEs in SBIs among COVID-19 patients cannot be overstated. However, there are certain limitations and important questions surrounding the delivery route of these phage-derived therapies and their impact on the host. This chapter underscores the importance of understanding the mechanisms and applications of PDEs in combating bacterial infections. By harnessing their potential, healthcare professionals can develop targeted interventions to mitigate the burden of SBIs and improve patient outcomes.

Author contributions

A.N. prepared the first draft of the manuscript. L.L., X.Z., Y.L. and Y.C. were responsible for this manuscript. All authors have read and agreed to the published version of the manuscript.

Funding

This study was funded by grants from the Natural Science Youth Foundation of Shandong Province (ZR2022QC028); the National Key Research and Development Project (2023YFE0107600); the Agricultural Scientific and Technological Innovation Project of Shandong Academy of Agricultural Sciences (CXGC2022E10; CXGC2023F10); the Innovation Capability Improvement Project for Science and Technology SMEs in Shandong Province (2022TSGC2384).

Conflicts of interest

There are no conflicts of interest.

Author details

Amina Nazir[1,2], Lulu Li[1,2], Xiaonan Zhao[1,2], Yuqing Liu[1,2] and Yibao Chen[1,2*]

1 Shandong Key Laboratory of Animal Disease Control and Breeding, Institute of Animal Science and Veterinary Medicine, Shandong Academy of Agricultural Sciences, P.R. China

2 Key Laboratory of Livestock and Poultry Multi-omics of MARA, P.R. China

*Address all correspondence to: yibaochen2012@126.com

References

[1] Shahin K, Zhang L, Mehraban MH, Collard J-M, Hedayatkhah A, Mansoorianfar M, et al. Clinical and experimental bacteriophage studies: Recommendations for possible approaches for standing against SARS-CoV-2. Microbial Pathogenesis. 2022:105442. DOI: 10.1016/j.micpath.2022.105442

[2] Feng Y, Ling Y, Bai T, Xie Y, Huang J, Li J, et al. COVID-19 with different severities: A multicenter study of clinical features. American Journal of Respiratory and Critical Care Medicine. 2020;**201**(11):1380-1388

[3] Kubin CJ, McConville TH, Dietz D, Zucker J, May M, Nelson B, et al. Characterization of bacterial and fungal infections in hospitalized patients with coronavirus disease 2019 and factors associated with health care-associated infections. Open forum. Infectious Diseases. 2021;**8**(6):ofab201. DOI: 10.1093/ofid/ofab201

[4] Vaillancourt M, Jorth P. The unrecognized threat of secondary bacterial infections with COVID-19. MBio. 2020;**11**(4):e01806-e01820

[5] Feldman C, Anderson R. The role of co-infections and secondary infections in patients with COVID-19. Pneumonia. 2021;**13**(1):1-15

[6] Catalano A, Iacopetta D, Ceramella J, Scumaci D, Giuzio F, Saturnino C, et al. Multidrug resistance (MDR): A widespread phenomenon in pharmacological therapies. Molecules. 2022;**27**(3):616. DOI: 10.3390/molecules27030616

[7] Nazir A, Ali A, Qing H, Tong Y. Emerging aspects of jumbo bacteriophages. Infection and Drug Resistance. 2021;**14**:5041

[8] Nazir A, Qi C, Shi N, Gao X, Feng Q, Qing H, et al. Characterization and genomic analysis of a novel Drexlervirial bacteriophage IME268 with lytic activity against Klebsiella pneumoniae. Infection and Drug Resistance. 2022;**15**:1533-1546. DOI: 10.2147/idr.s347110

[9] Nazir A, Dong Z, Liu J, Zhang X, Tahir RA, Ashraf N, et al. Sequence analysis of a jumbo bacteriophage, Xoo-sp14, that infects Xanthomonas oryzae pv. Oryzae. Microbiology Resource Announcements. 2020;**9**(48):e01072-e01020

[10] Nazir A, Dong Z, Liu J, Tahir RA, Rasheed M, Qing H, et al. Genomic analysis of bacteriophage Xoo-sp13 infecting Xanthomonas oryzae pv. Oryzae. Archives of Virology. 2021;**166**(4):1263-1265

[11] Nazir A, Dong Z, Liu J, Tahir RA, Ashraf N, Qing H, et al. Isolation, characterization, and genome sequence analysis of a novel lytic phage, Xoo-sp15 infecting Xanthomonas oryzae pv. Oryzae. Current Microbiology. 2021;**78**(8):3192-3200

[12] Chen Y, Wang S, Wang Y, Zhangxiang L, Chen H, Li X, et al. Complete genome sequence of the novel phage vB_EcoS_PHB17, which infects Shiga-toxin-producing Escherichia coli. Archives of Virology. 2019;**164**(12):3111-3113

[13] Wu N, Dai J, Guo M, Li J, Zhou X, Li F, et al. Pre-optimized phage therapy on secondary. Acinetobacter baumannii infection in four critical

COVID-19 patients. 2021;**10**(1):612-618. DOI: 10.1080/22221751.2021.1902754

[14] Wu N, Chen L-K, Zhu T. Phage therapy for secondary bacterial infections with COVID-19. Current Opinion in Virology. 2022;**52**:9-14. DOI: 10.1016/j.coviro.2021.11.001

[15] Olszak T, Shneider MM, Latka A, Maciejewska B, Browning C, Sycheva LV, et al. The O-specific polysaccharide lyase from the phage LKA1 tailspike reduces pseudomonas virulence. Scientific Reports. 2017;**7**(1):1-14

[16] Nazir A, Song J, Chen Y, Liu Y. Phage-derived Depolymerase: Its possible role for secondary bacterial infections in COVID-19 patients. Microorganisms. 2023;**11**(2):424

[17] Azeredo J, García P, Drulis-Kawa Z. Targeting biofilms using phages and their enzymes. Current Opinion in Biotechnology. 2021;**68**:251-261. DOI: 10.1016/j.copbio.2021.02.002

[18] Abdelrahman F, Easwaran M, Daramola OI, Ragab S, Lynch S, Oduselu TJ, et al. Phage-encoded endolysins. Antibiotics. 2021;**10**(2):124

[19] Lin H, Paff ML, Molineux IJ, Bull JJ. Antibiotic therapy using phage Depolymerases: Robustness across a range of conditions. Viruses. 2018;**10**(11):E622. DOI: 10.3390/v10110622

[20] Chen Y, Sun E, Yang L, Song J, Wu B. Therapeutic application of bacteriophage PHB02 and its putative depolymerase against Pasteurella multocida capsular type a in mice. Frontiers in Microbiology. 2018;**9**:1678

[21] Zhang Q, Bastard P, Bolze A, Jouanguy E, Zhang S-Y, Effort CHG, et al. Life-threatening COVID-19: Defective interferons unleash excessive inflammation. Med (N Y). 2020;**1**(1):14-20. DOI: 10.1016/j.medj.2020.12.001

[22] Manohar P, Loh B, Nachimuthu R, Hua X, Welburn SC, Leptihn S. Secondary bacterial infections in patients with viral pneumonia. Frontiers in Medicine. 2020;**7**:420

[23] Farrell JM, Zhao CY, Tarquinio KM, Brown SP. Causes and consequences of COVID-19-associated bacterial infections. Frontiers in Microbiology. 2021;**12**:682571. DOI: 10.3389/fmicb.2021.682571

[24] Hendaus MA, Jomha FA. Covid-19 induced superimposed bacterial infection. Journal of Biomolecular Structure and Dynamics. 2021;**39**(11):4185-4191

[25] Mumcuoğlu İ, Çağlar H, Erdem D, Aypak A, Gün P, Kurşun Ş, et al. Secondary bacterial infections of the respiratory tract in COVID-19 patients. Journal of Infection in Developing Countries. 2022;**16**(7):1131-1137. DOI: 10.3855/jidc.16724

[26] DeVoe C, Segal MR, Wang L, Stanley K, Madera S, Fan J, et al. Increased rates of secondary bacterial infections, including enterococcus bacteremia, in patients hospitalized with coronavirus disease 2019 (COVID-19). Infection Control and Hospital Epidemiology. 2022;**43**(10):1416-1423. DOI: 10.1017/ice.2021.391

[27] Zahariadis G, Gooley TA, Ryall P, Hutchinson C, Latchford MI, Fearon MA, et al. Risk of ruling out severe acute respiratory syndrome by ruling in another diagnosis: Variable incidence of atypical bacteria coinfection based on diagnostic assays. Canadian Respiratory Journal. 2006;**13**(1):17-22

[28] Chertow DS, Memoli MJ. Bacterial coinfection in influenza: A grand rounds review. JAMA. 2013;**309**(3):275-282

[29] Zhou F, Yu T, Du R, Fan G, Liu Y, Liu Z, et al. Clinical course and risk factors for mortality of adult inpatients with COVID-19 in Wuhan, China: A retrospective cohort study. The Lancet. 2020;**395**(10229):1054-1062

[30] Dadashi M, Khaleghnejad S, Abedi Elkhichi P, Goudarzi M, Goudarzi H, Taghavi A, et al. COVID-19 and influenza Co-infection: A systematic review and meta-analysis. Frontiers in Medicine. 2021;**8**:681469. DOI: 10.3389/fmed.2021.681469

[31] Bai Y, Tao X. Comparison of COVID-19 and influenza characteristics. Journal of Zhejiang University. Science. B. 2021;**22**(2):87-98. DOI: 10.1631/jzus.b2000479

[32] Vijay S, Bansal N, Rao BK, Veeraraghavan B, Rodrigues C, Wattal C, et al. Secondary infections in hospitalized COVID-19 patients: Indian experience. Infection and Drug Resistance. 2021;**14**:1893

[33] Bahceci I, Yildiz IE, Duran OF, Soztanaci US, Harbawi ZK, Senol FF, et al. Secondary bacterial infection rates among patients with COVID-19. Cureus. 2022;**14**(2):e22363

[34] De Bruyn A, Verellen S, Bruckers L, Geebelen L, Callebaut I, De Pauw I, et al. Secondary infection in COVID-19 critically ill patients: A retrospective single-center evaluation. BMC Infectious Diseases. 2022;**22**(1):1-7

[35] Shafran N, Shafran I, Ben-Zvi H, Sofer S, Sheena L, Krause I, et al. Secondary bacterial infection in COVID-19 patients is a stronger predictor for death compared to influenza patients. Scientific Reports. 2021;**11**(1):1-8

[36] Zhang H, Zhang Y, Wu J, Li Y, Zhou X, Li X, et al. Risks and features of secondary infections in severe and critical ill COVID-19 patients. Emerging Microbes & Infections. 2020;**9**(1):1958-1964

[37] Pawar RD, Balaji L, Mehta S, Cole A, Liu X, Peradze N, et al. Viral load and disease severity in COVID-19. Internal and Emergency Medicine. 2022;**17**(2):359-367. DOI: 10.1007/s11739-021-02786-w

[38] Rigoni M, Torri E, Nollo G, Donne LD, Rizzardo S, Lenzi L, et al. "Long COVID" results after hospitalization for SARS-CoV-2 infection. Scientific Reports. 2022;**12**(1):9581. DOI: 10.1038/s41598-022-13077-5

[39] Knight GM, Glover RE, McQuaid CF, Olaru ID, Gallandat K, Leclerc QJ, et al. Antimicrobial resistance and COVID-19: Intersections and implications. eLife. 2021;**10**:e64139. DOI: 10.7554/elife.64139

[40] Rangel K, Chagas TPG, De-Simone SG. Acinetobacter baumannii infections in times of COVID-19 pandemic. Pathogens. 2021;**10**(8):1006. DOI: 10.3390/pathogens10081006

[41] Qu J, Cai Z, Liu Y, Duan X, Han S, Liu J, et al. Persistent bacterial coinfection of a COVID-19 patient caused by a genetically adapted Pseudomonas aeruginosa chronic colonizer. Frontiers in Cellular and Infection Microbiology. 2021;**11**:641920. DOI: 10.3389/fcimb.2021.641920

[42] Taglialegna A. Reviving colistin. Nature Reviews Microbiology. 2023;**21**(7):411-411. DOI: 10.1038/s41579-023-00907-0

[43] Jamilloux Y, Henry T, Belot A, Viel S, Fauter M, El Jammal T, et al. Should we stimulate or suppress immune responses in COVID-19? Cytokine and anti-cytokine interventions. Autoimmunity reviews. 2020;**19**(7):102567. DOI: 10.1016/j.autrev.2020.102567

[44] Tian W, Zhang N, Jin R, Feng Y, Wang S, Gao S, et al. Immune suppression in the early stage of COVID-19 disease. Nature Communications. 2020;**11**(1):5859. DOI: 10.1038/s41467-020-19706-9

[45] Rouyer M, Strazzulla A, Youbong T, Tarteret P, Pitsch A, de Pontfarcy A, et al. Ventilator-associated pneumonia in COVID-19 patients: A retrospective cohort study. Antibiotics (Basel). 2021;**10**(8):988. DOI: 10.3390/antibiotics10080988

[46] Maes M, Higginson E, Pereira-Dias J, Curran MD, Parmar S, Khokhar F, et al. Ventilator-associated pneumonia in critically ill patients with COVID-19. Critical Care. 2021;**25**(1):25. DOI: 10.1186/s13054-021-03460-5

[47] Wang B, Zhang L, Wang Y, Dai T, Qin Z, Zhou F, et al. Alterations in microbiota of patients with COVID-19: Potential mechanisms and therapeutic interventions. Signal Transduction and Targeted Therapy. 2022;**7**(1):143. DOI: 10.1038/s41392-022-00986-0

[48] Hernández-Terán A, Mejía-Nepomuceno F, Herrera MT, Barreto O, García E, Castillejos M, et al. Dysbiosis and structural disruption of the respiratory microbiota in COVID-19 patients with severe and fatal outcomes. Scientific Reports. 2021;**11**(1):21297. DOI: 10.1038/s41598-021-00851-0

[49] Elezkurtaj S, Greuel S, Ihlow J, Michaelis EG, Bischoff P, Kunze CA, et al. Causes of death and comorbidities in hospitalized patients with COVID-19. Scientific Reports. 2021;**11**(1):4263. DOI: 10.1038/s41598-021-82862-5

[50] Callender LA, Curran M, Bates SM, Mairesse M, Weigandt J, Betts CJ. The impact of pre-existing comorbidities and therapeutic interventions on COVID-19. Frontiers in Immunology. 2020;**11**:1991. DOI: 10.3389/fimmu.2020.01991

[51] Nguyen D, Jeon H-M, Lee J. Tissue factor links inflammation, thrombosis, and senescence in COVID-19. Scientific Reports. 2022;**12**(1):19842. DOI: 10.1038/s41598-022-23950-y

[52] Lewis K. Platforms for antibiotic discovery. Nature Reviews Drug Discovery. 2013;**12**(5):371-387

[53] Drulis-Kawa Z, Majkowska-Skrobek G, Maciejewska B. Bacteriophages and phage-derived proteins–application approaches. Current Medicinal Chemistry. 2015;**22**(14):1757-1773

[54] Abedon ST, García P, Mullany P, Aminov R. Phage Therapy: Past, Present and Future. Vol. 8. Lausanne, Switzerland: Frontiers Media SA; 2017

[55] Silver LL. Challenges of antibacterial discovery. Clinical Microbiology Reviews. 2011;**24**(1):71-109

[56] Weber-Dąbrowska B, Jończyk-Matysiak E, Żaczek M, Łobocka M, Łusiak-Szelachowska M, Górski A. Bacteriophage procurement for therapeutic purposes. Frontiers in Microbiology. 2016;7:1177

[57] Rahman MU, Wang W, Sun Q, Shah JA, Li C, Sun Y, et al. Endolysin, a promising solution against antimicrobial resistance. Antibiotics (Basel). 2021;**10**(11):1277. DOI: 10.3390/antibiotics10111277

[58] Latka A, Maciejewska B, Majkowska-Skrobek G, Briers Y, Drulis-Kawa Z. Bacteriophage-encoded virion-associated enzymes to overcome the carbohydrate barriers during the infection process. Applied Microbiology and Biotechnology. 2017;**101**(8):3103-3119

[59] Maciejewska B, Olszak T, Drulis-Kawa Z. Applications of bacteriophages versus phage enzymes to combat and cure bacterial infections: An ambitious and also a realistic application? Applied Microbiology and Biotechnology. 2018;**102**(6):2563-2581

[60] Tian F, Li J, Nazir A, Tong Y. Bacteriophage—A promising alternative measure for bacterial biofilm control. Infection and Drug Resistance. 2021;**14**:205

[61] Mann NH. The potential of phages to prevent MRSA infections. Research in Microbiology. 2008;**159**(5):400-405. DOI: 10.1016/j.resmic.2008.04.003

[62] Loeffler JM, Fischetti VA. Synergistic lethal effect of a combination of phage lytic enzymes with different activities on penicillin-sensitive and -resistant Streptococcus pneumoniae strains. Antimicrobial Agents and Chemotherapy. 2003;**47**(1):375-377. DOI: 10.1128/aac.47.1.375-377.2003

[63] Schmelcher M, Donovan DM, Loessner MJ. Bacteriophage endolysins as novel antimicrobials. Future Microbiology. 2012;**7**(10):1147-1171

[64] Voorhees PJ, Cruz-Teran C, Edelstein J, Lai SK. Challenges & opportunities for phage-based in situ microbiome engineering in the gut. Journal of Controlled Release. 2020;**326**:106-119. DOI: 10.1016/j.jconrel.2020.06.016

[65] Ho MKY, Zhang P, Chen X, Xia J, Leung SSY. Bacteriophage endolysins against gram-positive bacteria—An overview on the clinical development and recent advances on the delivery and formulation strategies. Critical Reviews in Microbiology. 2022;**48**(3):303-326

[66] Pires DP, Oliveira H, Melo LDR, Sillankorva S, Azeredo J. Bacteriophage-encoded depolymerases: Their diversity and biotechnological applications. Applied Microbiology and Biotechnology. 2016;**100**(5):2141-2151. DOI: 10.1007/s00253-015-7247-0

[67] Kim S, Jin JS, Choi YJ, Kim J. LysSAP26—A new recombinant phage endolysin with a broad spectrum antibacterial activity. Viruses. 2020;**12**(11):1340. DOI: 10.3390/v12111340

[68] Bae JY, Jun KI, Kang CK, Song KH, Choe PG, Bang JH, et al. Efficacy of intranasal administration of the recombinant endolysin SAL200 in a lethal murine Staphylococcus aureus pneumonia model. Antimicrobial Agents and Chemotherapy. 2019;**63**(4):e02009-18. Published 2019 Mar 27. DOI: 10.1128/AAC.02009-18

[69] Zelmer A, Martin MJ, Gundogdu O, Birchenough G, Lever R, Wren BW, et al. Administration of capsule-selective endosialidase E minimizes upregulation of organ gene expression induced by experimental systemic infection with Escherichia coli K1. Microbiology (Reading, England). 2010;**156**(Pt 7):2205

[70] Waseh S, Hanifi-Moghaddam P, Coleman R, Masotti M, Ryan S, Foss M, et al. Orally administered P22 phage tailspike protein reduces salmonella colonization in chickens: Prospects of a novel therapy against bacterial infections. PLoS One. 2010;**5**(11):e13904

[71] Wu M, Hu K, Xie Y, Liu Y, Mu D, Guo H, et al. A novel phage PD-6A3, and its Endolysin Ply6A3, with extended lytic activity against Acinetobacter baumannii. Frontiers in Microbiology. 2018;**9**:3302. DOI: 10.3389/fmicb.2018.03302

[72] Pan Y-J, Lin T-L, Chen C-C, Tsai Y-T, Cheng Y-H, Chen Y-Y, et al. Klebsiella phage ΦK64-1 encodes multiple depolymerases for multiple host capsular types. Journal of Virology. 2017;**91**(6):e02457-e02416

[73] Yuan Y, Li X, Wang L, et al. The endolysin of the Acinetobacter baumannii phage vB_AbaP_D2 shows broad antibacterial activity. Microbial Biotechnology. 2021;**14**(2):403-418. DOI: 10.1111/1751-7915.13594

[74] V. Volozhantsev N, M. Shpirt A, I. Borzilov A, et al. Characterization and therapeutic potential of bacteriophage-encoded polysaccharide Depolymerases with β galactosidase activity against Klebsiella pneumoniae K57 capsular type. Antibiotics. 2020;**9**(11):732

[75] Chen X, Liu M, Zhang P, Xu M, Yuan W, Bian L, et al. Phage-derived Depolymerase as an antibiotic adjuvant against multidrug-resistant Acinetobacter baumannii. Frontiers in Microbiology. 2022;**13**:845500. DOI: 10.3389/fmicb.2022.845500

[76] Liu Y, Mi Z, Mi L, Huang Y, Li P, Liu H, et al. Identification and characterization of capsule depolymerase Dpo48 from Acinetobacter baumannii phage IME200. PeerJ. 2019;7:e6173

[77] Rice CJ, Kelly SA, O'Brien SC, Melaugh EM, Ganacias JC, Chai ZH, et al. Novel phage-derived depolymerase with activity against Proteus mirabilis biofilms. Microorganisms. 2021;**9**(10):2172

[78] Vasina DV, Antonova NP, Grigoriev IV, Yakimakha VS, Lendel AM, Nikiforova MA, et al. Discovering the potentials of four phage endolysins to combat gram-negative infections. Frontiers in Microbiology. 2021;**12**:748718. DOI: 10.3389/fmicb.2021.748718

[79] Furfaro LL, Payne MS, Chang BJ. Bacteriophage therapy: Clinical trials and regulatory hurdles. Frontiers in Cellular and Infection Microbiology. 2018;**8**:376. DOI: 10.3389/fcimb.2018.00376

[80] Pirnay J-P, Blasdel BG, Bretaudeau L, Buckling A, Chanishvili N, Clark JR, et al. Quality and safety requirements for sustainable phage therapy products. Pharmaceutical Research. 2015;**32**(7):2173-2179

[81] García R, Latz S, Romero J, Higuera G, García K, Bastías R. Bacteriophage production models: An overview. Frontiers in Microbiology. 2019;**10**:1187

Chapter 7

SARS-CoV-2 (COVID-19) Variants in Mexico

Luis Ulises Pérez-Arenas, Jessica Paola Plascencia-Roldán, Guadalupe Irazú Morales-Reyes, Gilberto Flores-Vargas, María de Jesús Gallardo-Luna, Efraín Navarro-Olivos, Francisco Javier Magos-Vázquez and Nicolás Padilla-Raygoza

Abstract

Coronavirus disease 2019 (COVID-19) is an infectious disease caused by the Severe Acute Respiratory Syndrome Coronavirus 2 (SARS-CoV-2). Due to the virus transmission and propagation since its origin, numerous mutations and variants have occurred. The concern relies on the ability to evade natural immunity and cause infections, even bypassing the immunity generated after the application of vaccines. The World Health Organization classified the variants into "variants of interest" (VOI) and "variants of concern" (VOC). From 2020 to 2021, the VOC variants were the alpha, beta, gamma, and delta types, currently adding the omicron variant. On the other hand, the VOI variants were the eta, iota, kappa, lambda, and mu types. The importance of their study leads to the problem of the possible generation of new waves of contagion, after their appearance, with a high possibility that the immunity known as herd achieved with some previous variant does not become effective.

Keywords: COVID-19, SARS-CoV-2 variants, SARS-CoV-2, spike glycoprotein, coronavirus

1. Introduction

The coronavirus disease 2019 (COVID-19) appeared at the end of 2019, and the virus causing the infection was named Severe Acute Respiratory Syndrome Coronavirus 2 (SARS-CoV-2) virus [1].

Coronaviruses come from the Nidovirales order, from the Coronaviridae family and Coronaviridae subfamily, and the latter includes four genera: alphacoronavirus, betacoronavirus, gammacoronavirus, and deltacoronavirus [2–4]. They infect both mammals (alpha and betacoronaviruses) and birds (gamma and delta coronaviruses) [4]. Currently, seven of them affect humans [5, 6].

Human coronaviruses (HCoV) have been identified for almost 50 years [7]. These are the alpha genus HCoV-229E, HCoV-NL63, and the betacoronavirus HCoV-OC43 and HCoV-HKU1 [8, 9]. The latest betacoronavirus found include the Severe Acute

Respiratory Syndrome Coronavirus (SARS-CoV) and the Middle East Respiratory Syndrome Coronavirus (MERS-CoV) [8, 9].

The SARS-CoV was identified in Guangdong, China. The reports indicate it spread to 29 countries between November 2002 and July 2003 [10, 11]. On the other hand, MERS-CoV received its name after being identified in Jeddah, Saudi Arabia, in 2012. The outbreak in the Arabian Peninsula reached 27 countries by April 2012 [11].

SARS-CoV and MERS-CoV are of zoonotic origin, and bats are considered the natural hosts, being highly pathogenic since they have caused epidemics of diseases in the last two decades [12–15].

A new infectious disease caused by a virus recently emerged; likewise, the first genomic sequencing data obtained from this virus did not match the previously sequenced coronaviruses, which indicated the existence of a new coronavirus strain (2019-nCoV) that was later assigned the specific name of SARS-CoV-2 [16, 17]. It was detected after the report of a group of patients with pneumonia of unknown etiology in December 2019 in Wuhan, Hubei, Province of China [18, 19]. Some of the first patients visited a wet shellfish market, where several other wildlife species were sold [19].

Due to the severity caused by this disease and likewise its high potential for worldwide spread, the World Health Organization (WHO) declared it a global health emergency on January 31, 2020 [17]. On February 11, 2020, the Coronaviridae Study Group of the International Committee on Virus Taxonomy named this new betacoronavirus SARS-CoV-2 [20]. On March 11, 2020, the WHO declared a pandemic state worldwide [17].

2. Structure and pathogenesis

SARS-CoV-2 is an enveloped virus with a single-stranded ribonucleic acid (RNA) genome of the beta-coronavirus genus. This RNA helps to encode mainly four structural proteins, these include the spike glycoprotein (S), which is one of the most important in the pathophysiological process; likewise, the envelope protein (E), membrane (M), and nucleocapsid (N); also, such as hemagglutinin esterase (HE) and among other 16 nonstructural proteins such as helicase and RNA-dependent RNA polymerase that help transcription and viral replication [21].

The spike protein (S) of SARS-CoV-2 is responsible for the entry of the virus into the host cell. It is divided by the enzyme furin, which results in two subunits, S1 and S2. The S1 subunit contains a region called the receptor-binding domain (RBD), which binds to the angiotensin-converting enzyme 2 (ACE-2) receptor and thus activates the host cell entry process. The RBD part is considered the main target of neutralizing antibodies after infection; in the same way, it is crucial for vaccine development or another therapeutic plan. On the other hand, in the S1 subunit, there is also a portion named the N-terminal domain (NTD), and it also plays a significant role in antigenicity [22].

The chief transmission mechanism is through the airway, direct contact with viral particles through flugge droplets when coughing, speaking, or sneezing; likewise, through aerosols or by direct contact. Therefore, the onset of the pathology lies with the interaction and fusion of the SARS-CoV-2 virus with the ACE-2 receptors that are mainly expressed in the lungs, allowing entry and, at the same time, the release of this viral RNA inside the cell. Then, the viral RNA initiates the translation of the viral proteins and, in turn, the replication of the genome at the cytoplasmic level, thus developing virions of the SARS-CoV-2 virus, which spread, making the respiratory tract the first line of infection and the virus entry. Therefore, it is the more affected system, resulting in the main respiratory manifestations [21]. The ACE-2 receptors are not only found in the respiratory system; they are widely expressed in the body in different tissues of the apparatus and systems, such as at the cardiovascular, gastrointestinal, and genitourinary levels, among others, leading the organism to show a mild disease to a multisystem compromise or death [2, 3, 21, 23].

There are four main phases in the pathogenic mechanism of COVID-19. These phases summarize the overall pathogenic mechanism of COVID-19, from the initial invasion to the long-term complications associated with the disease [24]. These are:

- Invasion: The SARS-CoV-2 virus uses receptors, such as ACE-2, to recognize and infect various cells, including those that do not express ACE2. It allows it to infect different types of cells in the body.

- Blockade of innate antiviral immunity: During this phase, the virus produces various structural and nonstructural proteins that block the ability of the innate immune system to fight infection. It allows the virus to replicate and evade the body's initial defenses.

- Activation of viral defense mechanisms: The virus develops mechanisms to evade and suppress the body's adaptive immune response. It implies passive and active virus protection in the inflammatory centers and continuous virus synthesis in the organism.

- Acute and long-term complications: At this stage, the virus can lead to the spread of variants and trigger acute and chronic complications associated with COVID-19. These complications can include the induction of autoimmune and autoinflammatory responses, as the generation of mechanisms that suppress the immune response and cause multisystem inflammation [24].

3. Evolution of the mutation of SARS-CoV-2 variants

Since the beginning of the COVID-19 outbreak and up to now, the SARS-CoV-2 virus has evolved and has produced some alarming variations. Although nowadays there is a high increase in both natural and vaccine-mediated immunity, many countries are still experiencing resurgences of COVID-19 disease due to the appearance of different and new variants of the SARS-CoV-2 [22].

We must remember and differentiate between *mutation*, *variant*, and *strain*, specifically in the context of the epidemiology of the SARS-CoV-2 virus:

- Mutation: Refers to the change in the virus's genetic sequence. For example, the D614G mutation is an aspartic acid substitution for glycine at position 614 of the virus spike glycoprotein.

- Variant: Used to describe genomes that differ in sequence from a reference genome. Nevertheless, this term is less precise since two variants can differ in one or several mutations.

- Strain: Strictly speaking, a variant is a strain when it shows a demonstrably different phenotype. It may include differences in terms of antigenicity (ability to be recognized by the immune system), transmissibility (ability to spread between individuals), or virulence (severity of the disease it causes) [25].

In summary, a mutation is a change in the genetic sequence, a variant is a genome that differs from a reference genome, and a strain is a variant that shows demonstrable phenotypic differences. These distinctions are important for understanding the epidemiology and characteristics of the SARS-CoV-2 virus.

Mutations often offer evolutionary benefits at the molecular level, such as increased recognition by the target cell, more effective entry into cells, or the ability to evade the immune system, tend to persist and can establish themselves in each virus lineage [26].

We refer to clinically and epidemiologically significant variants as those that, due to one or more mutations, can evade natural immunity and cause reinfections, evade immunity generated after vaccination and cause infections in vaccinated persons, evade the effectiveness of treatments such as antivirals, monoclonal antibodies, and convalescent plasma; on the other hand, they influence the severity of the disease with greater virulence, alter the transmission dynamics with a greater capacity to infect, and affect the accuracy of diagnostic tests [27].

RNA viruses, such as coronaviruses, come to present a considerably higher evolution rate than DNA viruses. The reason is its high susceptibility to replication errors caused by RNA polymerase or reverse transcriptase; furthermore, the higher viral population and its rapid replication rate also contribute to this accelerated evolutionary process [24, 28]. Although viruses commonly have a high mutation rate, SARS-CoV-2 has an enzyme – the RNA-dependent RNA polymerase – able to correct mistakes. This feature could explain why SARS-CoV-2 has a lower mutation rate than other RNA viruses [27]. However, the mutations that manage to emerge depend on a process of natural selection: only those that give the virus greater transmission capacity or the ability to evade the immune system persist in the population. Genetic analysis of the virus at the epidemiological level allows us to observe this evolution [27].

4. New variants and their nomenclature

As SARS-CoV-2 has been transmitted and spread, numerous mutations and variants have occurred. Over time, these have emerged and, in turn, have been organized and classified [27]. Given their classifications, the genetic changes of the virus, the increase in the speed of contagion, and aggressiveness are considered, besides the reduction in the effectiveness of public health measures, diagnoses, vaccines, and available treatments [26].

The UK Institute of Public Health has its own terminology, calling variants of concern those having a significant epidemiological impact. They also use the term Variants Under Investigation (VUI) to refer to those that can become variants of concern (VOC). The United States Centers for Disease Control (CDC) and Prevention and the World Health Organization (WHO) have adopted the definition of "variants of care" and have introduced the term "variants of interest" (VOI) -with an interpretation equivalent to VUI- and recommend its use globally [27].

In June 2020, the WHO Task Force on Viral Evolution was established, specifically focused on SARS-CoV-2 variants, their phenotype, and their impact on control measures. This group later became the Technical Advisory Group on the Evolution of the SARS-CoV-2 Virus. At the end of 2020, with the appearance of variants that represented a greater risk to public health worldwide, the WHO began to characterize some of them as VOI and VOC with the aim of the objective of setting priorities in surveillance and research globally and guiding the response to COVID-19. In May 2021, WHO began assigning simple, easy-to-pronounce names to main variants. In March 2023, WHO updated its surveillance system and working definitions for variants of concern, variants of interest, and variants under monitoring (VUM) [29].

5. SARS-CoV-2 variants

5.1 Alpha (B.1.1.7)

In the United Kingdom, in December 2020, the detection of a new variant of the SARS-CoV-2 virus, known as B.1.1.7 according to the Pango lineage nomenclature system, was reported. The WHO designated it the alpha variant. It was the first VOC identified. Retrospective analysis revealed that this VOC was already in circulation in September 2020 in the UK. The B.1.1.7 lineage spread rapidly in the UK and became the predominant variant in early 2021. It has subsequently spread successfully to most European countries. As of November 2021, local transmissions of this lineage have been recorded in 175 countries [30].

In Mexico, the B.1.1.7 lineage was identified for the first time in December 2020. Since then, a gradual increase in its circulation frequency was observed, reaching its peak in May 2021, but without becoming the predominant variant [30].

The data suggests that this variant is between 43% and 90% more contagious than previously existing lineages in the UK. Concerning the severity of the disease, although some reports have not shown clear evidence of an increase in mortality associated with the alpha variant, others have shown its connection with more severe diseases [22].

5.2 Beta (B.1.351)

The beta VOC variant shows three RBD mutations (N501Y, E484K, and K417N), as well as some NTD mutations, except for the 69/70 deletion. It was identified in South Africa in October 2020, and cases have since been detected elsewhere outside South Africa. There is no conclusive evidence to suggest increased mortality associated with this variant. Nevertheless, some reports indicate that the E484K mutation may affect neutralization by various monoclonal antibodies, including casirivimab, bamlanivimab, and etesevimab. In addition, the beta variant has shown higher resistance to the neutralizing activity of convalescent plasma and sera from individuals immunized with the mRNA-1273, BNT162b2, and AZD1222 vaccines [22, 28].

5.3 Gamma (P.1)

RBD mutations were detected in the gamma variant, which was cataloged as VOC. On January 6, 2021, the gamma variant was identified in four Japanese citizens who arrived in Tokyo after traveling to the Amazonian region of Brazil a few days earlier. This variant caused an increase in infection in the Manaus region of Brazil, where most of the population had already been infected by SARS-CoV-2. This variant is associated with increased transmissibility, risks of reinfection, and mortality. Like the beta variant, the gamma variant shows resistance to neutralization by various monoclonal antibodies, convalescent plasma, and vaccine sera [22, 28, 31].

5.4 Delta (B.1.617.2)

The delta variant, a VOC, was identified in India in early 2021. This variant exhibits the L452R mutation in the RBD and the P681 mutation in the furin cleavage site. In addition, it has several additional mutations in the spike protein (T19R, R158G, T478K, and D950N), as mutations in the orf3, orf7a, and nucleocapsid genes. The delta variant quickly displaced the alpha variant in multiple countries and became the dominant VOC globally. The delta variant has increased transmissibility due to possible mechanisms such as a higher infectious viral load, a longer virus shedding duration, and a higher reinfection rate due to antibody escape. The susceptibility of the delta variant to convalescent plasma and the sera of persons vaccinated with BNT162b2 and AZD1222 is reduced. Nevertheless, one study showed that BNT162b2 offers higher protection against the delta variant than AZD1222. In addition, the delta variant can resist bamlanivimab and some other monoclonal antibodies (mAbs) [22, 28, 31].

5.5 Omicron (B.1.1.529)

The omicron variant of the SARS-CoV-2 virus was first detected in South Africa in November 2021 and has spread to more than 50 countries. Omicron has different subvariants, BA.1 being the most transmissible and globally dominant, displacing the delta variant. BA.2 then emerged and replaced BA.1 in some countries. In addition, other subvariants such as BA.4/5 and BA.2.12.1 have been identified, which have a higher transmission capacity than BA.2 [22].

Omicron has more than 30 mutations in its spike proteins, some of which can affect the sites where antibodies bind to neutralize the virus. These subvariants have shared mutations, such as E484, K417N, T478K, N501Y, and P681H, associated with increased transmissibility and antibody evasion. However, each subvariant also has unique mutations [22].

Studies have shown a decreased ability of vaccine and convalescent sera to neutralize omicron subvariant BA.1. However, sera from persons vaccinated with boosters or previously infected showed antibodies that can still neutralize BA.1. The efficacy of vaccinations and boosters is similar for BA.1 and BA.2 [22, 32].

Limited cross-reactions have been observed between the different subvariants of omicron and other coronaviruses. Some therapeutic monoclonal antibodies, such as bamlanivimab, imdevimab, casirivimab, and etesevimab, have decreased efficacy against omicron subvariants. However, sotrovimab maintains some activity, albeit reduced, against BA.2, BA.4/5, and BA.2.12.1. Other monoclonal antibodies, such as tixagevimab/cilgavimab and adintrevimab, are partially active against BA.2 and BA.4/5 [22, 33].

In summary, the omicron variant of SARS-CoV-2 has generated different subvariants with mutations in spike proteins, which may affect the neutralization capacity of antibodies. Even as vaccines and therapeutic antibodies show less efficacy against omicron, boosters, and prior infection may provide only some protection against the identified subvariants.

6. Epidemiology of COVID-19 in Mexico

The global impact caused by the pandemic has been uneven in different parts of the world. Latin America has experienced a high impact due to the disease, presenting higher mortality rates than Western European countries. Mexico has been especially vulnerable due to underlying risk factors in its population, such as cardiovascular diseases such as dyslipidemia, hypertension, and type 2 diabetes. This combination of factors has generated greater severity, where poverty and limiting social factors, such as access to medical care, have been determining factors in the epidemiological outcome [26].

In May 2020, a mutation in the SARS-CoV-2 spike protein known as D614G occurred, which became prevalent in virus genomes worldwide. This mutation gave rise to lineage B – named as in the Pango nomenclature – which has remained the predominant lineage in the phylogenetic landscape. This lineage presents a greater infection capacity, competitiveness, viral load, and transmission in human and animal models. So far, five main VOCs have been identified at different stages of the pandemic in Mexico; alpha, beta, gamma, delta, and omicron. However, the omicron lineage is the most dominant, presenting more than 50 mutations, of which more than 30 are in the spike (S) protein [26].

In the last update on the epidemiology of COVID-19 in Mexico at the national level, updated in July 2023, published by the General Directorate of Epidemiology, 7,633,355 confirmed cumulative cases were reported. The distribution by sex of the confirmed cases was 53.66% for women and 46.34% for men. The general hospitalization percentage was 9.57%. The most frequent and chief comorbidities are hypertension at 11.90%, obesity at 9.59%, diabetes at 8.74%, and finally smoking at 5.41% [34].

On the other hand, in negative cases, a total of 11,638,267 have been registered. In suspected cases with a total of 830,243, recovered cases with 6,885,378, and active cases with 3558 [34].

7. SARS-CoV-2 (COVID-19) variants in Mexico

Despite the constant work against COVID-19 in the public health and research context, there have been severe resurgences in the number of cases, where the different variants of the virus are currently found, with the omicron variant predominating. Keeping infected people isolated from the onset of symptoms is one of the best alternatives since scientific findings suggest a shorter transmission and incubation period than other variants [35]. Over time, all kinds of information have changed because all viruses change with time, as does SARS-CoV-2, the virus that causes COVID-19 [29].

Although the COVID-19 pandemic began at the end of 2019 and the beginning of 2020, the Mexican government, through the Secretary of Health of Mexico, began the analysis and specific report of the genomic surveillance of the SARS-CoV-2 virus in Mexico's National and State Distribution of variants since August 30, 2021, and which is currently under development and in constant updating report [35].

From 2020 to 2021, the VOC variants were classified with the alpha, beta, gamma, and delta types; while, to the VOI variants with the eta, iota, kappa, lambda, and mu types. Besides, the genomic analysis in Mexico during 2020–2021 COVID-19 was documented through the global exchange initiative from genomic surveillance data for influenza viruses and SARS-CoV-2 (GISAID). Until October 18, 2021, up to epidemiological week 40, 32,081 sequences were reported [35].

The WHO classification of the variants was maintained early in 2022. Nevertheless, at the same time, a different variant named "omicron" was identified. Therefore, during the year, the omicron variant was classified as VOC with its respective classification with Subvariants of omicron under monitoring (from November 20, 2022) BA.5, BA.2.75, BA.4.6, XBB, and BA.2.3.20. VOI and VUM were maintained and, as additional data, the variants BQ.1, BW.1, and DL.1 were reported in this type [35].

In turn, during the year 2022, there was a high difference between the beginning and the end of the year. From April 4, 2022, to December 30, 2022, the reported sequences by GISAID increased from 57,823 to 81,429 [35].

Regarding 2023, from January 16, 2023, to May 4, 2023, the number of sequences reported by the GISAID increased from 81,914 to 87,447 [35].

Table 1 shows the information published through the global initiative for sharing data on the GISAID. It is worth mentioning that, for greater understanding, the VUM reports were excluded since they are constantly modified daily. The order by prevalence in 2021 is the following: delta, gamma, alpha, and beta. During 2022, the most prevalent VOCs were delta, with 25,434, followed by omicron, with 23,681. On the other hand, during 2023, the only predominant VOC was omicron, with a total of 34,499. The only exception added as a VOI was the last reported on May 4, 2023, because a type of lineage descendants of omicron reported as XBB.1.5 and XBB.1.16.

Year Date	Kind of variants	Variant name	Total National from each variant
From August 30 to October 18, 2021	VOC	Alpha	1759
		Beta	19
		Gamma	2711
		Delta	12,697
From April 4 to December 30, 2022	VOC	Delta	25,434
		Omicron	23,681
From January 16 to May 4, 2023	VOC	Omicron	34,499
From May 4 to June 30, 2023	VOI	Omicron (XBB.1.5)	1032
		Omicron (XBB.1.16)	1
Total			101,833

VOC: Variants of Concern, VOI: Variants of Interest.
Source: With data obtained from the public database GISAID https://www.gisaid.org/

Table 1.
Summary of the evolution of the variants of concern of COVID-19 in Mexico.

8. Epidemiological impact

The mutation D614G was identified in January 2020. Two months later, it came to present greater infectivity. In June, it became the predominant one in the world. Currently, 100% of the active variants have this mutation [27]. Thus, the importance of the impact of these variants and the possible generation of new waves of contagion. After their appearance, the immunity achieved with some previous variants could not be effective [27].

9. Vaccines and new variants

As we continue to learn more about this new virus, it remains an unprecedented event in world history [36]. The emergence of the pandemic led to the discovery of ways to achieve herd immunity and reduce the harmful effects of COVID-19 through vaccines. Remembering that the development of vaccines must go hand in hand with genomic surveillance [27]. Nowadays, these efforts have shown valuable results and are under implementation in all nations. Because it was necessary to synthesize the evidence of the effectiveness of vaccines against VOCs of SARS-CoV-2, various studies were carried out [36].

Baoqi Zeng et al. [37] conducted several pieces of research, including randomized controlled trials (RCTs), cohort studies, and case-control studies that evaluated vaccine effectiveness over our continuing-study variants of concern (alpha, beta, gamma, delta, or omicron), making a cut until March 4, 2022.

The variants of concern have mutations in their spike protein. Zeng B et al. [37] found that the complete vaccination of the COVID-19 vaccines was effective against the alpha, beta, gamma, delta, and omicron variants, with an effectiveness of 88.0, 73.0, 63.0, 77.8, and 55.9%, respectively. Also, it was found that the delta and omicron variants presented 95.5 and 80.8%, respectively, of effectiveness with the booster dose. Finally, mRNA vaccines (BNT162b2 or mRNA-1273) have higher effectiveness against variants of concern than other vaccines [37].

In other in vitro studies involving the Pfizer and AstraZeneca vaccines, decreased antibody titers against the delta variant were shown [27].

10. Signs and symptoms of COVID-19

The signs reported by individuals suffering from COVID-19 differ between those experiencing mild symptoms and those facing more severe illness. Symptoms can appear within 2 to 14 days after contact with the virus. Symptoms can vary in intensity, from mildly to severely [38, 39].

The most common symptoms of COVID-19 are the following:

- Fever
- Shaking chills
- Sore throat

Other accompanying symptoms:

- Muscle pain
- Severe fatigue or tiredness
- Severe runny, stuffy nose, or sneezing
- Headache
- Eye pain
- Dizziness
- New and persistent cough
- Tightness or pain in the chest
- Respiratory distress
- Hoarsely
- Numbness or tingling
- Nausea, vomiting, abdominal pain/stomachache, or diarrhea
- Loss of appetite
- Loss or change of taste or smell
- Difficulty breathing.

Symptoms of severe illness from COVID-19 and needing urgent medical attention include:

- Difficulty breathing, especially at rest, or an inability to speak in full sentences.
- Confusion
- Drowsiness or unconsciousness
- Persistent pain or pressure in the chest
- Cold or clammy skin or pale or bluish skin
- Loss of speech or mobility.

This previous enumeration does not cover all the possible signs. Symptoms may change their presentation with new variants of COVID-19 and may differ depending on vaccination status. The CDC continually updates this list as more COVID-19

Wave	Predominant variants	Confirmed cases	Case fatality rate (%)	Hospitalizations (%)	Clinical data predominant
First (March to September 2020)	B.1, B.1.1, B.1.1.222	809,387	12.3	25.1	Headache Fever Myalgia Arthralgia General malaise Odynophagia
Second (September 2020 to April 2021)	B1.1.222 B.1.1.519	1,538,110	8.7%	16.4%	Headache Fever Odynophagia Myalgia Arthralgia
Third (November 2021 to March 2022)	Alpha Delta Gamma	1,439,463	4.2	9.8	Cough Fever, Headache Rhinorrhea Odynophagia
Fourth (December 2021 to March 2022)	Omicron BA.1	1,722,625	1.2	3.4	Cough Headache Fever Odynophagia Rhinorrhea

Source: Taken from [40].

Table 2.
Waves of COVID-19 in Mexico (March 2020–March 2022) by predominant variants and clinical data.

information piles up. Older people and those with preexisting conditions such as heart disease, lung disease, or diabetes are at higher risk of experiencing severe complications from COVID-19 [38, 39].

Regarding Mexico, Loza A. et al. [40] reported four waves of COVID-19 from March 2020 to March 2022. **Table 2** shows the data about the predominant variants, the clinical manifestations, and figures about hospitalization and deaths. It is noted that hospitalization decreased with each wave, and so did the case fatality rate.

11. Conclusion

SARS-CoV-2 has generated different variants. These variants have been characterized as having specific genetic changes that may affect their transmissibility, disease severity, response to vaccines, and available treatments. Some variant has been shown to be more transmissible than the original strain of the virus and has raised global concerns due to their ability to spread rapidly.

The study of new SARS-CoV-2 variants supports the public health efforts for COVID-19 pandemic containment. It provides valuable information about the possible consequences of new scenarios. It is important to note that besides transmissibility, clinical manifestations play a crucial role in assessing the potential impact of new SARS-CoV-2 variants since they can cause a significant strain on health services. In the case of Mexico, the number of cases grew, but the CFR and the percentage of hospitalizations were lower in each successive wave driven by the predominant variants.

Finally, COVID-19 is a subject of active and constantly evolving research. Nowadays, additional research is underway to understand all the mechanisms involved and thus develop more effective and specific treatments. Although there is currently high natural and vaccine-mediated immunity, outbreaks continue to occur in some countries due to the different and constant variants of SARS-CoV-2.

Funding

None to the review.
The University Autonomous of Guadalajara will support the Open Access fee.

Conflict of interest

The authors declare no conflict of interest.

Author details

Luis Ulises Pérez-Arenas[1], Jessica Paola Plascencia-Roldán[2,3], Guadalupe Irazú Morales-Reyes[2,4], Gilberto Flores-Vargas[2], María de Jesús Gallardo-Luna[2], Efraín Navarro-Olivos[5], Francisco Javier Magos-Vázquez[5] and Nicolás Padilla-Raygoza[2*]

1 School of Medicine, Division of Health Sciences, University Autonomous of Guadalajara, Mexico

2 Department of Research and Technological Development, Directorate of Teaching and Research, Institute of Public Health from Guanajuato State, Guanajuato, México

3 Division of Health Sciences, Campus León, University of Guanajuato, León, México

4 School of Medicine, University Quetzalcoatl, Irapuato, México

5 Institute of Public Health from Guanajuato State, México

*Address all correspondence to: npadillar@guanajuato.gob.mx

References

[1] Guan WJ, Ni ZY, Hu Y, Liang WH, Ou CQ, He JX, et al. Clinical characteristics of coronavirus disease 2019 in China. The New England Journal of Medicine. 2020;**382**(18):1708-1720. DOI: 10.1056/NEJMoa2002032

[2] Chen Y, Liu Q, Guo D. Emerging coronaviruses: Genome structure, replication, and pathogenesis. Journal of Medical Virology. 2020;**92**(4):418-423. DOI: 10.1002/jmv.25681

[3] Lefkowitz EJ, Dempsey DM, Hendrickson RC, Orton RJ, Siddell SG, Smith DB. Virus taxonomy: The database of the international committee on taxonomy of viruses (ICTV). Nucleic Acids Research. 2018;**46**(D1):D708-D717. DOI: 10.1093/nar/gkx932

[4] Cui J, Li F, Shi ZL. Origin and evolution of pathogenic coronaviruses. Nature Reviews. Microbiology. 2019;**17**(3):181-192. DOI: 10.1038/s41579-018-0118-9

[5] Zhu N, Zhang D, Wang W, Li X, Yang B, Song J, et al. A novel coronavirus from patients with pneumonia in China, 2019. The New England Journal of Medicine. 2020;**382**(8):727-733. DOI: 10.1056/NEJMoa2001017

[6] International Committee on Taxonomy of Viruses Executive Committee. The new scope of virus taxonomy: Partitioning the virosphere into 15 hierarchical ranks. Nature Microbiology. 2020;**5**(5):668-674. DOI: 10.1038/s41564-020-0709-x

[7] Zhang SF, Tuo JL, Huang XB, Zhu X, Zhang DM, Zhou K, et al. Epidemiology characteristics of human coronaviruses in patients with respiratory infection symptoms and phylogenetic analysis of HCoV-OC43 during 2010-2015 in Guangzhou. PLoS One. 2018;**13**(1):e0191789. DOI: 10.1371/journal.pone.0191789

[8] Lim YX, Ng YL, Tam JP, Liu DX. Human coronaviruses: A review of virus-host interactions. Diseases. 2016;**4**(3):26. DOI: 10.3390/diseases4030026

[9] Zumla A, Chan JF, Azhar EI, Hui DS, Yuen KY. Coronaviruses - drug discovery and therapeutic options. Nature Reviews. Drug Discovery. 2016;**15**(5):327-347. DOI: 10.1038/nrd.2015.37

[10] Luk HKH, Li X, Fung J, Lau SKP, Woo PCY. Molecular epidemiology, evolution and phylogeny of SARS coronavirus. Infection, Genetics and Evolution. 2019;**71**:21-30. DOI: 10.1016/j.meegid.2019.03.001

[11] Park S. Epidemiology, virology, and clinical features of severe acute respiratory syndrome -coronavirus-2 (SARS-CoV-2; coronavirus Disease-19). Clinical and Experimental Pediatrics. 2020;**63**(4):119-124. DOI: 10.3345/cep.2020.00493

[12] Fehr AR, Perlman S. Coronaviruses: An overview of their replication and pathogenesis. Methods in Molecular Biology. 2015;**1282**:1-23. DOI: 10.1007/978-1-4939-2438-7_1

[13] de Wit E, van Doremalen N, Falzarano D, Munster VJ. SARS and MERS: Recent insights into emerging coronaviruses. Nature Reviews. Microbiology. 2016;**14**(8):523-534. DOI: 10.1038/nrmicro.2016.81

[14] Wong ACP, Li X, Lau SKP, Woo PCY. Global epidemiology of bat

coronaviruses. Viruses. 2019;**11**(2):174. DOI: 10.3390/v11020174

[15] Ye ZW, Yuan S, Yuen KS, Fung SY, Chan CP, Jin DY. Zoonotic origins of human coronaviruses. International Journal of Biological Sciences. 2020;**16**(10):1686-1697. DOI: 10.7150/ijbs.45472

[16] Zhu H, Wei L, Niu P. The novel coronavirus outbreak in Wuhan, China. Global Health Research and Policy. 2020;**5**:6. DOI: 10.1186/s41256-020-00135-6

[17] Dhama K, Khan S, Tiwari R, Sircar S, Bhat S, Malik YS, et al. Coronavirus disease 2019-COVID-19. Clinical Microbiology Reviews. 2020;**33**(4):e00028-e00020. DOI: 10.1128/CMR.00028-20

[18] Dos Santos WG. Natural history of COVID-19 and current knowledge on treatment therapeutic options. Biomedicine & Pharmacotherapy. 2020;**129**:110493. DOI: 10.1016/j.biopha.2020.110493

[19] Sun J, He WT, Wang L, Lai A, Ji X, Zhai X, et al. COVID-19: Epidemiology, evolution, and cross-disciplinary perspectives. Trends in Molecular Medicine. 2020;**26**(5):483-495. DOI: 10.1016/j.molmed.2020.02.008

[20] Machhi J, Herskovitz J, Senan AM, Dutta D, Nath B, Oleynikov MD, et al. The natural history, pathobiology, and clinical manifestations of SARS-CoV-2 infections. Journal of Neuroimmune Pharmacology. 2020;**15**(3):359-386. DOI: 10.1007/s11481-020-09944-5

[21] Morales Fernández JA, Wong Chew RM. Generalidades, aspectos clínicos y de prevención sobre COVID-19: México y Latinoamérica. Universitas Medica. 2021;**62**(3). DOI: 10.11144/Javeriana.umed 62-3.gacp. Available from: https://revistas.javeriana.edu.co/index.php/vnimedica/article/view/33065/25767

[22] Chen KK, Tsung-Ning Huang D, Huang LM. SARS-CoV-2 variants - evolution, spike protein, and vaccines. Biomedical Journal. 2022;**45**(4):573-579. DOI: 10.1016/j.bj.2022.04.006

[23] Tan W, Aboulhosn J. The cardiovascular burden of coronavirus disease 2019 (COVID-19) with a focus on congenital heart disease. International Journal of Cardiology. 2020;**309**:70-77. DOI: 10.1016/j.ijcard.2020.03.063

[24] Gusev E, Sarapultsev A, Solomatina L, Chereshnev V. SARS-CoV-2-specific immune response and the pathogenesis of COVID-19. International Journal of Molecular Sciences. 2022;**23**(3):1716. DOI: 10.3390/ijms23031716

[25] Lauring AS, Hodcroft EB. Genetic variants of SARS-CoV-2-what do they mean? Journal of the American Medical Association. 2021;**325**(6):529-531. DOI: 10.1001/jama.2020.27124

[26] García-López R, Laresgoiti-Servitje E, Lemus-Martin R, Sanchez-Flores A, Sanders-Velez C. The new SARS-CoV-2 variants and their epidemiological impact in Mexico. MBio. 2022;**13**(5):e0106021. DOI: 10.1128/mbio.01060-21

[27] Bedoya-Sommerkamp M, Medina-Ranilla J, Chau-Rodríguez V, Li-Soldevilla R, Vera Albújar Á, García PJ. Variantes del SARS-CoV-2: epidemiología, fisiopatología y la importancia de las vacunas. Revista Peruana de Medicina Experimental y Salud Pública. 2020;**38**(3):442-451. DOI: 10.17843/rpmesp.2021.383.8734

[28] Zhang Y, Zhang H, Zhang W. SARS-CoV-2 variants, immune escape, and countermeasures. Frontiers in Medicine. 2022;**16**(2):196-207. DOI: 10.1007/s11684-021-0906-x

[29] World Health Organization. Tracking SARS-CoV-2 variants. Available from: https://www.who.int/activities/tracking-SARS-CoV-2-variants/tracking-SARS-CoV-2-variants

[30] Zárate S, Taboada B, Muñoz-Medina JE, Iša P, Sanchez-Flores A, Boukadida C, et al. The alpha variant (B.1.1.7) of SARS-CoV-2 failed to become dominant in Mexico. Microbiology spectrum [Internet]. 2022;**10**(2):e0224021. DOI: 10.1128/spectrum.02240-21

[31] Zhou Z, Zhu Y, Chu M. Role of COVID-19 vaccines in SARS-CoV-2 variants. Frontiers in Immunology. 2022;**13**:898192. DOI: 10.3389/fimmu.2022.898192

[32] Rössler A, Knabl L, von Laer D, Kimpel J. Neutralization profile after recovery from SARS-CoV-2 omicron infection. The New England Journal of Medicine. 2022;**386**(18):1764-1766. DOI: 10.1056/NEJMc2201607

[33] Yamasoba D, Kosugi Y, Kimura I, Fujita S, Uriu K, Ito J, et al. Genotype to phenotype Japan (G2P-Japan) consortium. Neutralisation sensitivity of SARS-CoV-2 omicron subvariants to therapeutic monoclonal antibodies. The Lancet Infectious Diseases. 2022;**22**(7):942-943. DOI: 10.1016/S1473-3099(22)00365-6

[34] COVID-19 tablero México. COVID-19 Tablero México. Available from: https://datos.covid-19.conacyt.mx/

[35] Gobierno de México. Variantes COVID-19. Available from: https://coronavirus.gob.mx/variantes-covid-19/

[36] Francis AI, Ghany S, Gilkes T, Umakanthan S. Review of COVID-19 vaccine subtypes, efficacy and geographical distributions. Postgraduate Medical Journal. 2022;**98**(1159):389-394. DOI: 10.1136/postgradmedj-2021-140654

[37] Zeng B, Gao L, Zhou Q, Yu K, Sun F. Effectiveness of COVID-19 vaccines against SARS-CoV-2 variants of concern: A systematic review and meta-analysis. BMC Medicine. 2022;**20**(1):200. DOI: 10.1186/s12916-022-02397-y

[38] Centers for Disease Control and Prevention. Symptoms of COVID-19. 2022. Available from: https://www.cdc.gov/coronavirus/2019-ncov/symptoms-testing/symptoms.html

[39] World Health Organization. Coronavirus disease (COVID-19). Available from: https://www.who.int/emergencies/diseases/novel-coronavirus-2019/question-and-answers-hub/q-a-detail/coronavirus-disease-covid-19

[40] Loza A, Wong-Chew RM, Jiménez-Corona ME, Zárate S, López S, Ciria R, et al. Two-year follow-up of the COVID-19 pandemic in Mexico. Frontiers in Public Health. 2022;**10**. DOI: 10.3389/fpubh.2022.1050673

Section 2

Specific Organ Effects and Treatment Principles

Chapter 8

Spontaneous Hemorrhage in COVID 19 Patients

Fuad Pašić

Abstract

Much has been said and known of the possible occurrence of thromboembolism in various organ systems as part of Covid 19. The following Chapter discusses spontaneous hemorrhage in Covid 19 cases. Comparably to potential thromboembolism, it is found in a lesser percentage of patients, yet with serious repercussions on outcomes in the treatment of Covid 19 patients suffering from spontaneous hemorrhage. The Chapter examines and weighs in on the most optimal approaches to diagnosis and treatment of spontaneous hemorrhage in Covid 19 infection.

Keywords: Covid 19, respiratory virus, spontaneous hemorrhage, serious repercussions, treatment

1. Introduction

COVID-19 is a multisystem disease that can affect any organ – from the lungs, through the brain, skin, kidneys, digestive and nervous systems – since SARS-CoV-2 coronavirus is not merely a respiratory virus, but also pleiotropic.

In some patients with SARS-CoV-2 coronavirus infection no symptoms are registered (asymptomatic form); it can, however, be manifested by mild problems with the upper respiratory tract, such as common cold, but also pneumonia of various degrees of severity (from mild to severe) to life-threatening. Covid 19 is a highly prothrombogenic disease. Much has been said and known of the possible occurrence of thromboembolism in various organ systems. The Chapter focuses on spontaneous hemorrhage found in Covid 19 patients. It is found in lesser percentage of patients, yet with serious repercussions on treatment outcomes.

1.1 Human population and infectious diseases throughout history

Over 8 billion people live on planet Earth. The human population shares its living space with multiple other species. The planet is overpopulated. Clearly, humans live side by side with countless other pathogenic organisms of microscopic size, such as viruses, bacteria, parasites, fungi or other unconventional agents. Common diseases are found both in humans and animals.

The emergence of new diseases with pandemic potential has become one of the global medical challenges. Our knowledge of such diseases, if any, is very limited

IntechOpen

initially, forcing us to learn to curb such diseases in the most effective way. Viral Covid 19 infection of 2019 is one such disease. At one time, Covid 19 pandemic literally brought to stop numerous processes and flows on planet Earth. It brought scare to human race on across the continents and regardless of the development level of the country where it was recorded. It took time to gather relevant data and optimal algorithms for the treatment of this new viral infection reaching pandemic proportions. It took a while for this "intelligent and insidious" virus to become familiar with the human species and vice versa.

According to the World Health Organization (WHO), around 75% of emerging diseases affecting human population in the last decade are caused by pathogenic organisms originating from animals or animal products. Zoonoses have been known for many centuries, with more than 200 described to date [1].

In its 2020 conclusion, the UN Expert Commission on Biological Diversity warns that "in absence of preventive strategies, pandemics will break out more often, spread faster, kill more people and affect the global economy with more unprecedented devastating effects".

According to estimates published in the Journal of Science, there are 1.7 million unknown viruses among mammals and birds, of which 540,000 to 850,000 can infect humans. There is evident space for further scientific research, including points of concern, such as the emergence of new unknown diseases, pandemics and the like. In the 20th century, smallpox epidemic alone accounts for 300 to 500 million deaths. Smallpox is believed to be responsible for the death of 10% of the human population over the last thousand years [2]. The Spanish flu pandemic broke out in 1918, killing 21.5 million according to most referenced literature. More recent additional research after looking at the data and registers of developing countries says that between 50 and 100 million died from the Spanish flu [3–5]. Plague was synonymous with disease, hardships and suffering. People died from the plague in terrible agony. The plague epidemic marked the entire period of the late Middle Ages and part of the early Middle Ages. It is been long since the plague disappeared from Europe, but it is still smoldering in hotspots around the world such as Asia, Africa, North and South America [6]. Dubbed as the queen of diseases, malaria has been known since ancient. Some believe that it is largely responsible for the downfall of the Roman Empire. In the 20th century alone, it accounts for between 150 and 300 million deaths. Malaria still affects 228 million in different parts of the world, with as many as 405,000 deaths, especially in the poorest countries [7]. Epidemic typhus is louse-born by sucking the blood of a patient in the rickettsemia phase. The largest known epidemic of typhus hit Napoleon's army during the Russian campaign, killing half a million [8].

According to the most recent data from the World Health Organization, one and a half million still die from tuberculosis in the world today, and about ten million fall ill every year [9]. Leprosy is one of the oldest and most terrible diseases affecting people, synonymous with stigma and discrimination due to large bodily deformations. It has been known since ancient times as 'death before death'. Despite therapy, it is still endemic in some countries. Annually, 200,000 new cases are diagnosed [10].

Syphilis has been a constant and unwanted companion of mankind for more than 400 years. Since its first emergence, syphilis has been a stigmatized, shameful disease. It affected the lives of millions in all walks of life. Epidemics of various diseases occurred during the 19th century were quite common. Here, cholera stands out, causing an exceptionally high mortality rate.

1.2 Human population and infectious diseases in the 21st century

In early 21st century, bird flu caused by the A/H5N1 virus subtype was recorded in Asia in 2003. During 2009, the so-called swine flu caused by the H1N1 influenza virus emerged. The disease began to spread human to human, rising to the level of pandemic. SARS-CoV appeared in China 21 years ago (2002), as a severe viral respiratory disease that can cause death of up to 15% of the infected. In 2012, a new global threat emerged in Saudi Arabia, a disease called MERS-CoV, causing severe respiratory illness. Although most patients are geographically associated with the Arabian Peninsula, MERS-CoV has also been detected in other parts of the world. In 2013, global concern grew over the emergence of the Ebola virus disease in West Africa. Millions were at risk, and thousands fell ill.

The above overview portrays a series of very serious and severe diseases leaving significant and profound consequences on the evolution and development of the human population. In philosophical terms, a war is being waged on planet Earth as to who the real ruler of our living space is. Logically, man as a 'rational being' should be the one running the processes on the planet Earth. But looking at the adaptability of animals and other species, bacteria, viruses and many other microscopic organisms show that humans are in no position to claim the title of 'genuine managers' or the main stakeholders of the planet Earth in full capacity. Old and new diseases with old and new causative agents have led to the emergence of more resistant and more adaptable disease causative agents. Finding the most adequate patterns in the treatment of old and emerging diseases has become a genuine medical challenge.

2. Covid 19 and hemorrhage

2.1 Coronaviruses

Coronaviruses (lat. corona: wreath, crown < Greek. κορώνη: curved or rounded eend of something, ring + virus), are a group of viruses from the Coronaviridae family. The viral particle is spherical in shape with a diameter of 120 to 160 nm, and the spiky transmembrane glycoprotein outgrowths on the envelope with a length of 12 to 24 nm resemble a crown. The genome consists of single-stranded positive RNA composed of 26 to 32 thousand nucleotides, which ranks coronaviruses among the RNA viruses with the largest genomes. The viral particle consists of four to six structural polypeptides, with four viral proteins: the so-called spike protein (S-protein), nucleocapsid protein (N), membrane protein (M) and envelope protein (E). The virus enters the cytoplasm of the host cell by fusion of the viral envelope and the cytoplasmic membrane, mediated by the S-protein. Coronaviruses are not newly discovered viruses, but come with their own history. These viruses were first described in the sixties of the last century, as the isolates of the HCoV-229E and HCoV-OC43 viruses, highly widespread and common around the world. They appear sporadically, seasonally and possibly in smaller epidemics in the winter, and lead to an acute febrile illness of the upper respiratory system much like a common cold.

2.2 Who are Covid 19 patients susceptible to develop thromboembolic complications

Most frequent patients include bed-ridden, elderly, adipose, male, patients previously suffering from thrombosis and cancer patients. They are also patients with other significant comorbidities and those who are hospitalized in the intensive care unit and have medium-severe and severe forms of Covid 19. In patients with thrombosis, blood coagulation is increased, there is damage to the endothelium of blood vessels by the SARS-CoV-2 virus itself and multiple inflammatory processes. In Covid 19, the activities of several blood clotting factors (factor VIII, von Willebrand factor, fibrinogen and D-dimer) are also elevated (**Figure 1**).

Axial HRCT images of a 38-year-old man with COVID-19 ARDS admitted to ICU at the same level, performed at different times: baseline scan (A) and 7-month follow-up (B). The baseline scan (A) shows typical imaging features indicative of severe COVID-19 pneumonia, including extensive bilateral parenchymal consolidations, mainly affecting the posterior regions of lower lobes, bilateral focal ground-glass opacities in the anterior regions and patchy consolidation, peripherally distributed, resembling pulmonary fibrosis. The 7-month scan (B) shows a complete resolution of the parenchymal consolidations and the apparent fibrotic abnormalities.

2.3 Covid 19 patients with spontaneous hemorrhage

According to data, hemorrhage-related complications in elderly patients on anticoagulant therapy are estimated at around 5%, with an incidence of spontaneous hematomas of around 0.6% [11]. In cases of formation of large hematomas with hemodynamic instability, the prognosis is poor with multiple failure and organ failure [12], reaching a mortality of 30 to 50% [13, 14]. It has been proven that the COVID-19 infection causes a disorder of hemostasis [15], with a procoagulant state. This has led to the inclusion of thromboprophylactic (anticoagulant) therapy in most treatment protocols. There are also studies related to heparin-induced thrombocytopenia [16, 17]. The rationale behind is that a certain number of patients develop kidney failure due to coronavirus infection. This results in a prolonged half-life of heparin, which then circulates longer in the plasma. All this leads to 'pseudo overdose',

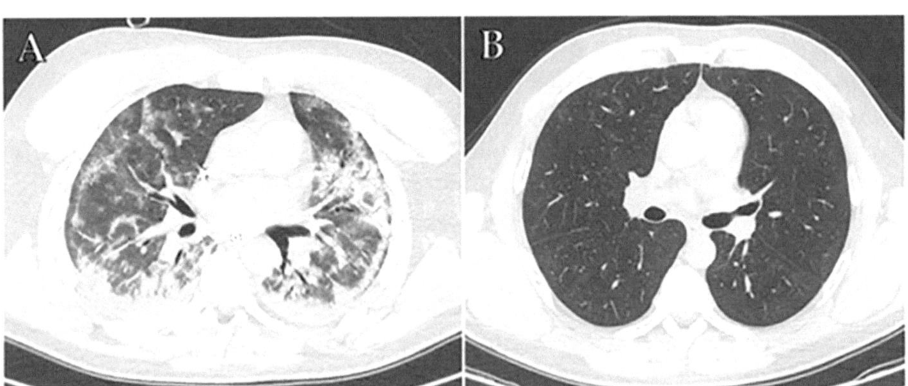

Figure 1.
Covid 19 pneumonia.

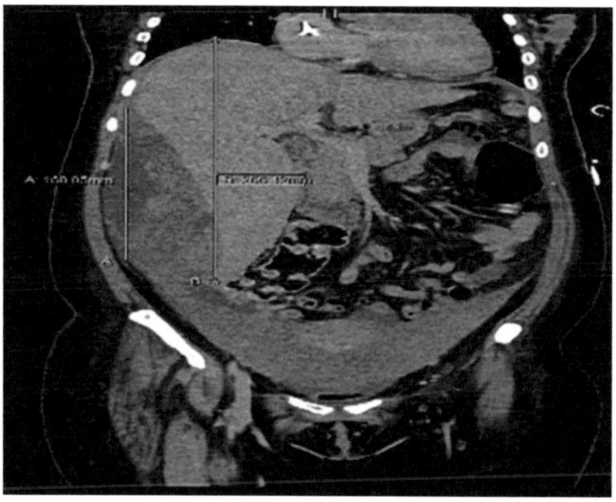

Figure 2.
Spontaneous hepatic hematoma as part of Covid 19.

increasing the risk of hemorrhage [18]. The incidence of hematoma in patients with COVID-19 due to coagulation disorders caused by the infection, together with thrombocytopenia due to heparin and overdose in patients with renal failure will be the subject of further research (**Figure 2**).

In patients with spontaneous hematoma or hemorrhage, (CT), computed tomography and (CT) angiography are absolutely needed and highly sensitive procedures to adequately diagnose the resulting hematomas, allowing for the size, location and artery responsible for the hemorrhage to be determined in full. It also identifies the location or vascular origin of hemorrhage in 95.2% of cases [19].

According to the available relevant papers, hemorrhages occurred in 2.22% of patients in the total number of those hospitalized with Covid 19 infection, that is, in 7.88% of the total number of patients hospitalized in ICU. Hemorrhage occurred in most cases in patients on anticoagulation, more so in men with multiple comorbidities, aged between 60 and 79 years. It mostly occurred in one anatomical region (especially retroperitoneal), with the most extensive hemorrhage in the chest wall [20]. This complication was diagnosed on average 16.7 days after admission and hospitalization. It occurred most often in severe forms of Covid 19 in patients who underwent invasive mechanical respiratory support, that is, cyclic pronation-supination measures. Hematomas were active in slightly less than half of the cases. The vast majority of patients were treated conservatively and survived [20].

COVID-19 is a highly prothrombogenic disease and therefore thromboprophylaxis is mandatory in hospitalized COVID-19 patients in order to improve treatment outcomes.

2.4 Thrombocytopenia

Zimmerman was the first to discover platelets in 1860, and their role in blood clotting was further elaborated in 1878 by Zimmerman and Hayran [21]. In short, platelets are essential for maintaining the integrity of the vascular endothelium and controlling bleeding from injury to small blood vessels through the formation of platelet plugs [22]. It is known thrombocytopenia is found in 2.5 percent of the normal population (**Table 1**) [23].

Mild: 100,000–150,000/μL
Moderate: 50,000–100,000/μL.
Severe: <50000/μL.

Table 1.
Classification of thrombocytopenia.

Thrombocytopenia is not a disease, but a diagnosis. Effective interpretation of thrombocytopenia requires gathering detailed information from the patient or the patient's family, followed by thorough examination and lab tests. Thrombocytopenia can occur with recently introduced new drugs or drugs taken only occasionally. Recent infections and previously diagnosed hematological diseases are mentioned as a possible reason for its occurrence. There are also non-hematological diseases that are known to reduce the number of platelets (eclampsia, sepsis, DIC, anaphylactic shock, hypothermia, massive transfusions). It is also found in cases of prior family history of hemorrhage, recent vaccination with live virus, in patients with poor nutritional status, pregnancy, recent organ transplantation from a donor sensitized to platelet alloantigens, and recent transfusion containing platelets in an allosensitized recipient. Possible alcohol consumption and risk factors for HIV should also be looked into. For asymptomatic patients with low platelet count, the physician should initially try to rule out artifactual or pseudothrombocytopenia as the etiology. Thrombocytopenia also requires that family history in terms of congenital thrombocytopenia is also looked at [24].

2.5 Thrombocytopenia and Covid 19

According to referenced literature, mild thrombocytopenia is present in 45 to 55% of patients positive for COVID-19 [25], but also, thrombocytopenia is found in 95% of patients with a severe form of Covid 19 infection [26]. Viral infection caused by Sars CoV-2 can vary from asymptomatic clinical forms to severe respiratory forms with acute respiratory distress. The hematopoietic system can also react to COVID-19 in several ways, from mild forms to life-threatening forms [27]. Moderate and severe forms of the disease can lead to the formation of thrombus and pulmonary embolism [25]. Usually, thrombocytopenia occurs 10 to 14 days after the onset of disease symptoms [28]. It becomes a potential biomarker of negative prognosis in COVID-19 patients [29]. The most frequently mentioned pathophysiological mechanism is that the SARS-CoV-2 virus causes hyperinflammation and hypercoagulability.

Risk factors for thrombocytopenia are older age, male, high APACHE II score, neutropenia, lymphopenia, elevated CRP and low PaO 2 /FiO 2 ratio. Thrombocytopenia can also be caused by a decrease in thrombopoietin (a regulator of megakaryopoiesis and platelet production) following hepatocyte damage in SARS-CoV-2 infection. In the bone marrow, viral infection of megakaryocytes can induce apoptosis and reduce platelet maturation. However, several cases have been presented in the medical literature showing that COVID-19 infection is associated with the onset or recurrence of immune thrombocytopenia (ITP), characterized by isolated thrombocytopenia, without any tendency to thrombosis [30]. Another possible interpretation is that the formed antibodies and immune complexes can enhance the removal of platelets in the circulation and that excessive activation of platelets can cause their increased removal in spleen and liver. Some patients may develop consumptive thrombocytopenia [30–32].

2.6 Coagulopathy in COVID-19

Development of consumptive coagulopathy (a blood clotting disorder in which coagulation factors and then platelets are consumed) is one of the most significant indicators of a poor outcome in COVID-19. An analysis of patients with COVID-19 pneumonia showed that abnormal coagulation tests at hospital admission were associated with a higher risk of death.

Here we have raised a real issue that requires additional efforts by doctors to understand these processes, since in consumptive coagulopathy or disseminated intravascular coagulation, there is simultaneously an increased risk of both hemorrhage and thrombosis, which is all associated with a high risk of fatal outcome in patients [33].

2.7 Guidelines for thromboprophylaxis in COVID-19

Numerous international medical associations have published recommendations on thromboprophylaxis for patients with COVID-19. Thus, the International Society on Thrombosis and Hemostasis (ISTH) notes that all hospitalized COVID-19 patients should receive medicinal thromboprophylaxis, the so-called low molecular weight heparin, unless suffering contraindications (for example, active hemorrhage or low platelet values - less than 25x109/L). Similar are the recommendations and guidelines of the American Society of Hematology (ASH), CHEST and ACC (American College of Cardiology) [34].

To highlight, if the patient is already on anticoagulant therapy for other reasons, the patient can continue with the existing chronic therapy unless contraindicated due to a change in the patient's clinical status (for example, the inability to administer drugs orally, developed an increased risk of hemorrhage, etc.). In such cases, the preference is to change the method of administration to low-molecular-weight heparin, administered as a subcutaneous injection.

2.8 Mechanism of spontaneous hemorrhage in Covid 19 patients

Covid 19 patients can develop spontaneous hemorrhage, but the mechanism of its occurrence has not yet been fully understood in all aspects. The most plausible explanation is that it is most likely due to a cascade of possible reasons that individually or combined cause the hemorrhage to occur. Coagulopathy, Cytokine storm, systematic inflammation, low platelet count, endothelitis with endothelial dysfunction, almost always accompanying cough associated with pneumonia with frequent changes in intratocacal and intra-abdominal pressure are some of the most frequently mentioned reasons for the occurrence of spontaneous hemorrhage in Covid 19 patients. Pronation maneuvers, treatment with anticoagulants, obesity, increased vascular sensitivity determined by a pro-inflammatory state, barotrauma from C-PAP ventilation, and cough with consequent increase in intra-abdominal pressure are among the risk factors for hemorrhage in patients with COVID- 19.

2.9 Who are the patients at risk for spontaneous hemorrhage?

It is important to detect patients who are at absolute risk of hemorrhage and for whom prescribed anticoagulant therapy may cause more harm than good. These are patients with DIC, thrombocytopenia, or previous hemorrhage tendencies. Patients who are already being treated for intracranial and genitourinary hemorrhages, epistaxis, and patients with tracheostomy should also be kept in mind.

2.10 Can we be more efficient in the detection and treatment of patients susceptible to spontaneous hemorrhage

Due care is needed in the projections of possible benefit and harm in patients with mild to moderate form of Covid 19 infection. Patients should be examined in the broader context of the patient's health.

It is imperative to detect patients at risk for hemorrhage by taking a very detailed history with detailed insight into the previous medical records of the patient with Covid 19.

Covid 19 can develop and manifest itself in several forms of illness (mild, medium and severe) but also in several variants with predominant symptoms (respiratory, gastrointestinal, neurological and other).

In a patient with Covid 19 with a moderate and severe form of infection, it is essential to consider a personalized modulated therapy with low molecular weight heparins, which will be optimized depending on the possible improvement or deterioration of the patient's general condition and health.

- Multidimensional assessment of the patient's condition will include the analysis of laboratory findings, blood count, renal parameters, inflammation parameters and assessment of the patient's general condition, especially in the period 10 to 14 days after hospitalization, as this is the time when the largest number of spontaneous hemorrhage occurs.

Several points to bear in mind in case of Covid 19 infection.

- It may not be possible to establish adequate contact with the patient.

- Concerned family and other accompanying members may not give all but only partial information about previous illnesses or if the patient is prone to hemorrhage.

- The patient but also the patient's family can be an important factor in obtaining relevant data essential for treatment. In the case of mass and other forms of illness, we need to simulate the most difficult scenarios and situations should be run.

Clinical situation in case.

The patient is in a very serious general condition on controlled mechanical ventilation with a severe Covid 19 form. The patient has family living in another city or country with no possibility of contact. It may be useful to reiterate:

If we already have a CT angio examination of a patient diagnosed with hemorrhage, clear information should be obtained on the following:

- Whether or not the patient is actively bleeding,

- Exact localisation, blood vessel, size of the bleed area, approximately calculated possible amount of blood in the hematoma,

- Run a clinical and biochemical assessment of the patient's condition,

Whether active treatment is required in a patient who is hemodynamically unstable. Assessment of methods to stop hemorrhage.

- Interventional radiology – Surgery

Preference is given to interventional radiology due to better results, faster and more effective targeted treatment of bleeding and faster overall recovery.

- In order to stratify and improve results and outcomes in treatment in a personalized approach to patients, medical professionals should have all fully functional and easily accessible IT tools at their disposal.

- Emerging diseases, unknown or partially known in their forms of manifestation, will require genuine commitment but also great knowledge of doctors and other medical workers in order to treat them successfully.

- The oft-repeated phrase of 'Personalized Medicine' will be in future tested in reality to see to what extent can we independently manage these new diseases that we have yet to become familiar with.

Speaking of spontaneous hemorrhage in narrow terms, the actual number of small or hidden hemorrhages can only be speculated. This area will need to be further defined. It is also important to say that there are several adopted revised protocols for the medical treatment of Covid 19 patients. What is common to all these protocols is the use of anticoagulants, which reduce the mortality rate.

3. Conclusion

Historical overview and analysis stand as a reminded that human population had been exposed to numerous mass diseases, pandemics and temptations accounting for hundreds of millions of lives. Some of these diseases have been largely eradicated, yet some are still smoldering with the emergence of bran new, utterly unexplored and fully undefined diseases.

More and more diseases noticeably originate from the same causative agents, affecting the health of both humans and animals, as well as other species with which we share the planet Earth.

Speaking of the Covid 19 pandemic, "we are still getting to know Covid 19 and the virus is getting to know the human population". We have gained loads of useful scientific knowledge about this disease, but the process is not fully finalized. In consideration of spontaneous hemorrhage as part of the Covid 19 infection, our activities should go along the lines how to improve the final outcomes in the treatment of this complication. It is very important to answer the following questions:

- How to prevent the possible hemorrhage.

- How to detect it timely and precisely.

- How to treat most adequately.

Spontaneous hemorrhage can be prevented by a well-trained doctor after conducting a solid interview, obtaining relevant anamnestic data and objectively interpreting the obtained laboratory findings. Mindful of all these elements gathered, a polymorphic disease such as Covid 19 will require dedicated medical professionals, personalized modulated therapy and optimized diagnostic and therapeutic treatment especially in patients at risk of hemorrhage.

Early or timely detection of a patient suffering from hemorrhage as part of the Covid 19 disease will be all the more complicated as it is most common in patients with severe forms of this disease. Repeated clinical examinations, the search for hidden areas of bleeding, more detailed monitoring of laboratory findings and the hemodynamic state of the patient will be a guarantee of better results.

Author details

Fuad Pašić
Department of General Abdominal Surgery, University Clinical Center Tuzla, Tuzla, Bosnia and Herzegovina

*Address all correspondence to: fuad.p@bih.net.ba; dr.fuadpasic@gmail.com; fuad.pasic@ukctuzla.ba

References

[1] World Health Organization (WHO). Available at: https://www.who.int/health-topics/ [Accessed April 11, 2020]

[2] Theves C, Biagini P, Crubezy E. The rediscovery of smallpox. Clinical Microbiology and Infection. 2014;**20**:210-218

[3] Morse SS. Emerging infections: Condemned to repeat? In: Relman DA, Hamburg MA, Choffnes RA, Mack A, editors. Microbial Evolution and Co-adaption: A Tribute to the Life and Scientific Legacies of Joshua Lederberg. Washington, DC: National Academies Press; 2009

[4] Taubenberger JK, Morens DM. 1918 influenza: The mother of all pandemics. Emerging Infectious Diseases. 2006;**12**:15-22

[5] Erkoreka A. Origins of the Spanish influenza pandemic (1918-1920) and its relation to the First World War. Journal of Molecular Genetic Medicine. 2009;**3**:190-194

[6] Cvetnić Ž. Kuga – bolest koja je promijenila svijet (I. dio). Vet. stn. 2014;**45**:85-95

[7] World Health Organization (WHO). Available at: https://www.who.int/health-topics/malaria [Accessed: April 11, 2020]

[8] Raoult D, Woodward T, Dumler S. The history of epidemic typhus. Infectious Disease Clinics of North America. 2004;**18**:127-140

[9] World Health Organization (WHO). Available at: https://www.who.int/health-topics/tuberculosis [Accessed: April 11, 2020]

[10] Visschedijk J, Van De Broek H, Eggense H, Lever P, Van Beers S, Klatser P. Review: Mycobacterium leprae – Millenium resistant! Leprosy control on the threshold of new era. Tropical Medicine & International Health. 2000;**5**:388-399

[11] Doham A, Darnige L, Sapoval M, Pellerin O. Spontaneous soft tissue hematomas. Diagn IntervImaging. 2015;**96**:789-796. DOI: 10.1016/j.diii.2015.03.014

[12] Bargellini I. Spontaneous bleedings in COVID-19 patients: An emerging complication. Cardiovascular and Interventional Radiology. 2020;**43**(7):1095-1096. DOI: 10.1007/s00270-020-02507

[13] Palumbo D, Guazzarotti G, De Cobelli F. Spontaneous major haemorrhage in covid-19 patients: Another brick in the wall of SARS-Cov-2-associated coagulation disorders? JVIR. 2020;**31**(9):148-150. DOI: 10.1016/j.jvir.2020.06.010

[14] Vergori A, Pianura E, Lorenzini P, Abramo A, et al. Spontaneous Ilio-psoas haematomas (IPHs): A warning for COVID-19 inpatients. Annals of Medicine. 2021;**53**(1):295-301

[15] Erdinc B, Raina JS. Spontaneous retroperitoneal bleed coincided with massive acute deep vein thrombosis as initial presentation of Covid-19. Cureus. 2020;**12**(8):e9772. DOI: 10.7759/cureus.9772

[16] Dorgalaleh A. Bleeding and bleeding risk in COVID-19. Seminars in Trombosis and Hemostasis. 2020;**46**(7):815-818. DOI: 10.1055/s-0040-1713434

[17] Lucatelli P, De Rubeis G, Citone M, Lucarelli NM, Pasqualini V, Sturiale M, et al. Heparin-related major bleeding in Covid-19-positive patient: Perspective from the outbreak. Cardiovascular and Interventional Radiology. 2020;**43**:1216-1217. DOI: 10.1007/s00270-020-02532-3

[18] Mattioli M, Benfaremo D, Fustini E, Gennarini S. Atypical spontaneuos haematomas in a patient with severe coronavirus disease 2019 (COVID-19). Seminars in Thrombosis and Hemostasis. 2020;**46**:856-858

[19] Nakamura H, Ouchi G, Miyagi K, Higure Y, Otsuki M, Nishiyama N, et al. Case report: Iliopsoas hematoma during the clinical course of severe COVID-19 in two male patients. The American Journal of Tropical Medicine and Hygiene. 2021;**104**(3):1018-1021

[20] Trentadue M, Calligaro P, Lazzarini G, Boseggia FB, Residori E, Hu J, et al. Spontaneous bleeding in COVID-19: A retrospective experience of an Italian COVID-19 hospital. SA Journal of Radiology. 2022;**26**(1):2509

[21] Levine SP. Thrombocytopenia: Pathophysiology and classification. In: Greer JP, Foerster J, Rodgers GM, Paraskevas F, Glader B, Arber DA, Means RT, editors. Wintrobe's Clinical Hematology. 12th ed. Philadelphia: Lippincott Williams & Wilkins Co.; 2009. pp. 1289-1334

[22] Consolini DM. Thrombocytopenia in infants and children. Pediatrics in Review. 2011;**32**(4):135-149

[23] Goldstein KH, Abramson N. Efficient diagnosis of thrombocytopenia. American Family Physician. 1996;**53**(3):915-920

[24] Sekhon SS, Roy V. Thrombocytopenia in adults: A practical approach to evaluation and management. Southern Medical Journal. 2006;**99**(5):491-498

[25] Helms J, Tacquard C, Severac F, Leonard-Lorant I, Ohana M, Delabranche X, et al. High risk of thrombosis in patients with severe SARS-CoV-2 infection: A multicenter prospective cohort study. Intensive Care Medicine. 2020;**46**:1089-1098

[26] Lippi G, Plebani M, Henry BM. Thrombocytopenia is associated with severe coronavirus disease 2019 (COVID-19) infections: A meta-analysis. Clinica Chimica Acta. 2020;**506**:145-148

[27] Wool GD, Miller JL. The impact of COVID-19 disease on platelets and coagulation. Pathobiology. 2021;**88**:15-27

[28] Xu XW, Wu XX, Jiang XG, Xu KJ, Ying LJ, Ma CL, et al. Clinical findings in a group of patients infected with the 2019 novel coronavirus (SARS-Cov-2) outside of Wuhan, China: Retrospective case series. BMJ. 2020;**368**:m606

[29] Zong X, Gu Y, Yu H, Li Z, Wang Y. Thrombocytopenia is associated with covid-19 severity and outcome: An updated meta-analysis of 5637 patients with multiple outcomes. Laboratoriums Medizin. 2021;**52**:10-15

[30] Tjendra Y, Al Mana AF, Espejo AP, Akgun Y, Millan NC, Gomez-Fernandez C, et al. Predicting disease severity and outcome in COVID-19 patients: A review of multiple biomarkers. Achieves in Pathology Lab Medicine. 2020;**144**:6. DOI: 10.5858/arpa.2020-0471-SA

[31] Pranata R, Lim MA, Yonas E, Huang I, Nasution SA, Setiati S, et al. Thrombocytopenia as a prognostic marker inCOVID-19 patients: Diagnostic test accuracy meta-analysis. Epidemiology Infections. 2021;**149**

[32] Liu Y, Sun W, Guo Y, Chen L, Zhang L, Zhao S, et al. Association between platelet parameters and mortality in coronavirus disease 2019: Retrospective cohort study. Platelets. 2020;**31**. DOI: 10.1080/09537104.2020.1754383

[33] Conway EM, Mackman N, Warren RQ, Wolberg AS, Mosnier LO, Campbell RA, et al. Understanding COVID-19-associated coagulopathy. Nature Reviews. Immunology. 2022;**22**(10):639-649

[34] Cuker A, Tseng EK, Nieuwlaat R, Angchaisuksiri P, Blair C, Dane K, et al. American Society of Hematology living guidelines on the use of anticoagulation for thromboprophylaxis in patients with COVID-19: January 2022 update on the use of therapeutic-intensity anticoagulation in acutely ill patients. Blood Advances. 2022;**6**(17):4915-4923

Chapter 9

Posterior Segment Ocular Findings in Critically Ill Patients with COVID

Rosa María Romero Castro, Gabriela González Cannata and Ana Sánchez Tlapalcoyoatl

Abstract

To describe ophthalmological fundoscopic findings in patients with COVID-19 admitted to the intensive care unit (ICU) of the largest third-level referral center for COVID-19 in Mexico City. In this cross-sectional single-center study, consecutive patients admitted to the ICU with a diagnosis of COVID-19 underwent fundus examination with an indirect ophthalmoscope. Clinical photographs were taken using a posterior-pole camera. We explored the association between ocular manifestations and demographic characteristics, inflammatory markers, hemodynamic factors, and comorbidities. Of 117 patients examined, 74 were male; the median age was 54 years (range: 45–63 years). Forty-two patients had ophthalmological manifestations (unilateral in 23 and bilateral in 19), and 10 of these patients had more than one ophthalmological manifestation. Ocular findings were papillitis (n = 13), cotton-wool spots (n = 12), retinal hemorrhages (n = 5), retinal nerve fiber layer edema (n = 8), macular whitening (n = 5), retinal vascular tortuosity (n = 4), papillophlebitis (n = 3), central retinal vein occlusion (n = 1), and branch retinal vein occlusion (n = 1). Ocular fundus manifestations were not associated with demographic characteristics, inflammatory markers, hemodynamic factors, or comorbidities. Over one-third of patients with severe COVID-19 had ophthalmological manifestations. The most frequent fundoscopic findings were optic nerve inflammation, microvasculature occlusion, and major vascular occlusions. We recommend long-term follow-up to prevent permanent ocular sequelae.

Keywords: chorioretinal vasculopathy, uveitis, retinal vein occlusion, optic neuritis, acute retinal ischemia, SARS-CoV-2, Covid-19, PAMM

1. Introduction

The COVID-19 pandemic was declared on March 11, 2020, by the World Health Organization (WHO). As is already known, the coronavirus belongs to the genus *Betacoronavirus* and the family Coronaviridae [1, 2].

The coronavirus causes a severe acute respiratory syndrome (SARS), which was responsible for the death of approximately 6,881,955 people worldwide, according to the Johns Hopkins University as of March 10, 2023 [3]. For the virus to enter human cells, it uses the angiotensin-converting enzyme 2 (ACE2), which is expressed in the lungs, heart, central nervous system (CNS), adrenal glands, and in the ocular globe. The structures that have this enzyme include the cornea, conjunctiva, sclera, ciliary body, retina, aqueous humor, vitreous humor, and iris [4, 5]. This explains the wide range of clinical manifestations that can occur in COVID-19 infection.

It has been found that the cluster of differentiation 147 (CD147) is expressed in the corneal and conjunctival epithelia and plays an important role in severe acute respiratory syndrome coronavirus 2 (SARS-CoV-2) infection [6], along with ACE2, which has been identified in the Müller cells of the retina, mainly in the inner nuclear layer [7], as well as in endothelial cells. This is where the theory of SARS-CoV-2 entry into the retina arises, which begins on the corneal and conjunctival surface and then spreads hematogenously to reach the choroid plexus, leading to the breakdown of the blood-retinal barrier mediated by CD147, facilitated by an inflammatory microenvironment [8–10].

The clinical findings of the anterior segment commonly described in COVID-19 infections occur in a range of 2–32% [11–13]. There are very few reports of posterior segment manifestations in hospitalized patients. A review of the literature showed a mean age of 47.4 ± 14.8 years [14], and ocular manifestations have been reported in 36% [15] of patients in the Intensive Care Unit (ICU) within a range of 4–55 days after the onset of the initial symptoms.

The exact role that SARS-CoV-2 plays in the retina during the infection is still not known for certain. Studies have been conducted using immunohistochemical analysis, where no RNA or spike protein was found in biopsies from deceased COVID-19 patients [16, 17]. On the other hand, Menuchin demonstrated in three-dimensional (3D) retinal tissue cultures, referred to as retinal organoids, evidence that SARS-CoV-2 can actively replicate in the retina [18].

2. Posterior segment ocular findings

2.1 Optic neuritis

The SARS-CoV induces neuronal death in the medullary respiratory center through the upregulation of inflammatory markers or through direct autophagy. The same hypothesis has been proposed for SARS-CoV-2, in which the virus infects a peripheral neuron and travels retrograde to the brain via synaptic transport [19].

The most common ocular finding reported by Romero [15] was inflammation of the optic nerve, including papillitis and papillophlebitis, in hospitalized patients. The reason why ganglion cells and the optic nerve are affected by COVID infection is explained by Menuchin's study [18] with retinal organoids, which suggests that the ganglion cell layer had a higher probability of being infected by SARS-CoV-2, up to 40%. It concluded that progenitor cells are less susceptible to infection than neurons. However, the pathophysiology is still not clear and may be related to vascular dysfunction caused by hypercoagulability or a process similar to viral infection-induced vasculitis in severely ill patients [20]. Neuro-ophthalmic manifestations in COVID-19 infection include optic neuritis, acute transverse myelitis, viral encephalitis, toxic encephalopathy, leukoencephalopathy, and acute disseminated encephalomyelitis [21].

Optic neuritis is defined as an inflammatory demyelinating condition that causes acute visual loss, generally monocular, and rarely binocular, very few cases of optic neuritis have been reported days after the onset of symptoms in patients with mild disease. Mechanisms responsible for these neuro-ophthalmic manifestations have been postulated, such as neurotropism and molecular mimicry, where viral antigens trigger a host immune response directed toward central nervous system myelin proteins [22, 23]. It can be associated with the spectrum of neuromyelitis optica, a disease associated with myelin oligodendrocyte glycoprotein [23], or infectious disease. The latter is more common in children, with common organisms being *Mycoplasma pneumoniae* and viruses, including SARS-CoV-2 [24].

Oculomotor paralysis of cranial nerves III, IV, or VI and VII [24–26] can result from direct viral infection or neurological complications, such as Guillain-Barré syndrome, Miller Fisher syndrome [27], or acute disseminated encephalomyelitis, and can occur in isolation or as polyneuropathies.

The prone position can cause anterior or posterior ischemic neuropathy, since this position has been shown to increase intraocular pressure to more than 40 mmHg [28]. On the other hand, this position has shown improved survival in patients with acute respiratory distress syndrome (ARDS) [29].

2.2 Retinal vascular occlusions

2.2.1 Central retinal vein occlusion (CRVO)

Central retinal vein occlusion (CRVO) is a common manifestation of the disease when it comes to posterior segment abnormalities. This was reported by Fonollosa, who found that 25 out of 35 patients presented with central retinal vein occlusion, and in some cases, it occurred bilaterally. CRVO occurs more frequently in the acute stages of COVID-19 infection, and it has been shown that it does not necessarily involve thrombotic and occlusive lesions in other organs but can be limited to the retina [30].

The involvement of retinal vasculature in COVID-19 infection can be explained by the state of hypercoagulability during the acute phase, leading to endothelial damage [31].

CRVO is characterized by painless visual loss accompanied by intraretinal hemorrhages in a flame-shaped pattern across the retinal surface, unlike branch retinal vein occlusion where hemorrhages are localized to the affected vessel's course. Other features may include cotton-wool spots and, in some cases, macular edema.

Risk factors associated with the development of CRVO include age over 50 years (in 90% of cases), systemic arterial hypertension, diabetes mellitus, and hyperlipidemia [32, 33]. These risk factors also predispose individuals to severe COVID-19 infection. In a large cohort of patients with a history of COVID-19 and CRVO, 68% of patients were under 40 years of age and had mild disease compared to the typical age of presentation. However, 36% of them had cardiovascular risk factors, and the procoagulant state during the acute phase of the disease increased the risk of ischemic events in this cohort [32, 33].

2.2.2 Central retinal artery occlusion (CRAO)

Thrombotic events in COVID-19 infection have been reported in 39% of patients [34]. Central retinal artery occlusion (CRAO) tends to develop frequently in patients during the acute phase of COVID-19 infection. For example, Acharya [35] reported the first case in a 60-year-old patient with acute respiratory distress syndrome, who had comorbidities, such as hypertension, dyslipidemia, stable coronary artery disease, and chronic obstructive pulmonary disease (COPD). After being placed on mechanical ventilation, the patient experienced sudden and painless vision loss, and ophthalmological examination revealed a cherry-red spot with retinal whitening.

While hypercoagulability is a leading cause of ischemic alterations, it's essential to recognize that this patient had comorbidities that increased the risk of such an event.

Macular whitening has also been reported as a finding in the posterior segment of hospitalized COVID-19 patients [15], likely due to cilioretinal artery hypoperfusion, believed to be secondary to vascular dysfunction caused by elevated levels of D-dimer, prothrombin, fibrinogen, partial thromboplastin time, and patient comorbidities such as hypertension and obesity.

2.3 Acute paracentral middle maculopathy (PAMM) and acute macular neuroretinopathy (NMA)

Acute paracentral middle maculopathy (PAMM) and acute macular neuroretinopathy (NMA) are caused by microvascular alterations in the deep retinal vessels [36–38].

Cases of concurrent NMA and PAMM with a COVID-19 diagnosis have been reported. Castro [37] reviewed the literature on reported cases and noted that all patients were under 55 years of age, predominantly female, without prior comorbidities, and that these conditions occurred 1 month after the diagnosis of SARS-CoV-2 infection as the sole systemic complication. These findings are significant because PAMM was previously known to predominantly occur in patients with cardiovascular risk factors [39].

A decrease in macular capillary density by 8% has been demonstrated in severe COVID-19 patients, as well as a decrease in the density of intermediate and deep retinal capillary plexuses in patients without previous comorbidities. There appears to be a correlation between the severity of the disease and the decrease in retinal vessel density [40].

2.4 Vascular alterations

The mechanism by which COVID-19 can affect retinal vasculature is still unknown, but several theories have been proposed. The angiotensin-converting enzyme 2 (ACE2) is believed to play a significant role in producing vasoconstriction, triggering thrombogenicity by increasing platelet and leukocyte adhesion [41]. It has been reported that COVID-19 infection can cause alterations in retinal microvasculature up to 8.86 times more [42].

Ivernizzi [43] evaluated the diameter of retinal veins 30 days after the onset of systemic symptoms and found that the diameter of both retinal veins and arteries was increased compared to the control group. Furthermore, the diameter was even larger in the more severe cases, leading to the conclusion that the dilation of retinal and pulmonary vessels could be secondary to increased blood supply due to the inflammatory response and endothelial damage. This theory about endothelial damage is supported by a study that observed decreased vessel density in the superficial capillary plexus, deep capillary plexus, and choriocapillaris, along with an increase in the foveal avascular zone, through optical coherence tomography (OCT) in a six-month follow-up after COVID-19 infection [44].

The use of retinal lesions as a biomarker for assessing the extent of COVID-19's impact on the brain has been proposed by de Figuereido [9]. This is based on theories about the mechanism of SARS-CoV-2 entry into the eye and its proximity to the central nervous system (**Figure 1**).

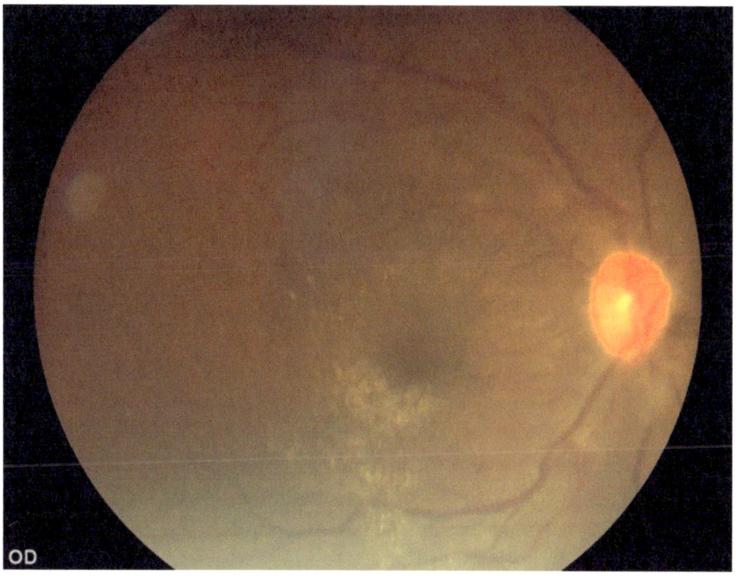

Figure 1.
Color fundus photograph showing tortuosity of vessels, hemorrhages in the temporal vascular arches and cottony exudates in the inferior temporal vascular arch with macular edema.

2.5 Vasculitis

Kawasaki-like [45] manifestations have been reported in association with COVID-19. The exact cause of this condition is still uncertain, but the most accepted theory is an aberrant immune response to a pathogen in genetically predisposed patients [46]. Endothelial cells can also be affected by COVID-19, leading to inflammation, apoptosis, and dysfunction [47].

There have been investigations regarding coronaviruses within the coronavirus family, such as the New Heaven virus identified in respiratory secretions of children with Kawasaki disease [48]. However, this finding has been highly debated, because the series of cases reported as Kawasaki-like has occurred in patients older than the usual age, with respiratory and gastrointestinal involvement, as well as meningeal and cardiovascular signs [46]. These clinical manifestations have also been reported in COVID patients, making it difficult to determine the exact etiology of these alterations.

Another form of vasculitis reported in the literature is seen in pediatric patients with chilblains and areas of vasculitis. Although no other abnormalities were found in these patients, vasculitis presentation is believed to be an autoimmune response in COVID-19 patients, possibly triggered by interferon type 1 (IFN), leading to acral skin lesions and vasculitis [49].

2.6 Retinal abnormalities

The exact route of SARS-CoV-2 infection to the retina is not known with certainty. It could occur through hematogenous dissemination or via nerve fibers through the optic nerve, potentially causing changes in the optic nerve and retina [21].

Cotton-wool spots have been reported in various series [15, 21, 50, 51] and have been referred to as retinal microangiopathy associated with COVID-19 [52]. These cotton-wool spots are not exclusive to COVID-19, as they have been observed in conditions like hypertension, human immunodeficiency virus (HIV) retinopathy [53], diabetic retinopathy [54], and giant cell arteritis [55]. Cotton-wool spots have been proposed as an indicator of some acute vascular event [56] or as a biomarker of systemic vascular disease [52]; however, imaging studies have not conclusively identified whether these cotton-wool spots are secondary to patients' comorbidities or simply the result of the treatments used [51].

However, cotton-wool spots have not only been reported in patients with severe illness. Landecho [52] and Pereira [56] observed these findings in asymptomatic patients 43 days after the onset of the first symptoms. The location can vary, either appearing on the surface of the retina or following the course of venous or arterial vessels.

In a study of hospitalized patients, cotton-wool spots, retinal nerve fiber layer edema, and retinal hemorrhages were the second most common ocular findings [15]. These findings are consistent with previous reports where flame hemorrhages were seen in 22.2% and peripheral retinal hemorrhages in 11.1% of severe patients [56] and support the hypothesis that the retinal tropism of SARS-CoV-2 is associated with the disruption of the blood-retinal barrier [9].

Zago [57] and Costa [36] reported the presence of localized white-yellowish points in the outer retina that were self-limiting and did not result in visual sequelae. Optical coherence tomography (OCT) revealed hyporeflectivity in the pigment epithelium of the retina and the ellipsoid layer, as well as a discontinuation of the outer segments of photoreceptors. Notably, these findings were observed in patients who had recovered from COVID-19 within an average time of 82 ± 36.4 days after the onset of their initial symptoms. Of this group, 51.5% had a severe disease course and 37.5% had a critical illness.

2.7 Choroidal abnormalities

It has been suggested that the retina and the choroid could be key sites for ocular infection due to the presence of angiotensin-converting enzyme, which is expressed in both the choroid and the retina. Among the observed changes, a decreased choroidal thickness has been reported in the subfoveal, temporal, and nasal quadrants in recovered patients without anticoagulant or antiplatelet therapy [58]. This is speculated to be linked to an exaggerated immune response during the early stages of the disease, leading to an increase in choroidal thickness [59], followed by a subsequent decrease due to endothelial damage, resulting in reduced choroidal thickness [60].

Irregular, wall-less dark holes among choroidal vessels have been reported in 21% of severe COVID-19 patients. These findings are similar to those seen in conditions like geographic atrophy and pachychoroid. These holes may represent a new drainage pathway for choroidal vessels through the lymphatic system or spaces filled with lipids that regulate the inflammatory process [61].

Author details

Rosa María Romero Castro*, Gabriela González Cannata
and Ana Sánchez Tlapalcoyoatl
Infectious Diseases Research Center, National Autonomous University of México,
Toluca, Mexico

*Address all correspondence to: rromerocastro@yahoo.com

References

[1] Chilamakuri R, Agarwal S. COVID-19: Characteristics and therapeutics. Cells [Internet]. 2021;**10**(2):206. DOI: 10.3390/cells10020206

[2] Sharma A, Ahmad Farouk I, Lal SK. COVID-19: A review on the novel coronavirus disease evolution, transmission, detection, control and prevention. Viruses [Internet]. 2021;**13**(2):202. DOI: 10.3390/v13020202

[3] COVID-19 map [Internet]. Johns Hopkins Coronavirus Resource Center. Available from: https://coronavirus.jhu.edu/map.html [Accessed: October 3, 2023]

[4] Yaguchi S, Ogawa Y, Shimmura S, Hatou S, Nakamura S, Inaba T, et al. Presence and physiologic function of the renin–angiotensin system in mouse lacrimal gland. Investigative Ophthalmology & Visual Science [Internet]. 2012;**53**(9):5416. DOI: 10.1167/iovs.12-9891

[5] Senanayake PD, Drazba J, Shadrach K, Milsted A, Rungger-Brandle E, Nishiyama K, et al. Angiotensin II and its receptor subtypes in the human retina. Investigative Ophthalmology & Visual Science [Internet]. 2007;**48**(7):3301-3311. DOI: 10.1167/iovs.06-1024

[6] Hamashima K, Gautam P, Lau KA, Khiong CW, Blenkinsop TA, Li H, et al. Potential modes of COVID-19 transmission from human eye revealed by single-cell atlas [internet]. bioRxiv. 2020. DOI: 10.1101/2020.05.09.085613

[7] Tikellis C, Johnston CI, Forbes JM, Burns WC, Thomas MC, Lew RA, et al. Identification of angiotensin converting enzyme 2 in the rodent retina. Current Eye Research [Internet]. 2004;**29**(6):419-427. DOI: 10.1080/02713680490517944

[8] Zhang Y, Stewart JM. Retinal and choroidal manifestations of COVID-19. Current Opinion in Ophthalmology [Internet]. 2021;**32**(6):536-540. DOI: 10.1097/icu.0000000000000801

[9] de Figueiredo CS, Raony Í, Giestal-de-Araujo E. SARS-CoV-2 targeting the retina: Host–virus interaction and possible mechanisms of viral tropism. Ocular Immunology and Inflammation [Internet]. 2020;**28**(8):1301-1304. DOI: 10.1080/09273948.2020.1799037

[10] Varga Z, Flammer AJ, Steiger P, Haberecker M, Andermatt R, Zinkernagel AS, et al. Endothelial cell infection and endotheliitis in COVID-19. Lancet [Internet]. 2020;**395**(10234):1417-1418. DOI: 10.1016/S0140-6736(20)30937-5

[11] Ulhaq ZS, Soraya GV. The prevalence of ophthalmic manifestations in COVID-19 and the diagnostic value of ocular tissue/fluid. Arbeitsphysiologie [Internet]. 2020;**258**(6):1351-1352. DOI: 10.1007/s00417-020-04695-8

[12] Zhou Y, Duan C, Zeng Y, Tong Y, Nie Y, Yang Y, et al. Ocular findings and proportion with conjunctival SARS-COV-2 in COVID-19 patients. Ophthalmology [Internet]. 2020;**127**(7):982-983. DOI: 10.1016/j.ophtha.2020.04.028

[13] Inomata T, Kitazawa K, Kuno T, Sung J, Nakamura M, Iwagami M, et al. Clinical and prodromal ocular symptoms in coronavirus disease: A systematic review and meta-analysis. Investigative Ophthalmology & Visual Science [Internet]. 2020;**61**(10):29. DOI: 10.1167/iovs.61.10.29

[14] Sen M, Honavar SG, Sharma N, Sachdev MS. COVID-19 and eye: A review of ophthalmic manifestations of COVID-19. Indian Journal of Ophthalmology [Internet]. 2021;**69**(3):488-509. DOI: 10.4103/ijo.IJO_297_21

[15] Romero-Castro RM, Ruiz-Cruz M, Alvarado-de la Barrera C, González-Cannata MG, Luna-Villalobos YA, García-Morales AK, et al. Posterior segment ocular findings in critically ill patients with covid-19. Retina [Internet]. 2022;**42**(4):628-633. DOI: 10.1097/iae.0000000000003457

[16] Casagrande M, Fitzek A, Spitzer M, Püschel K, Glatzel M, Krasemann S, et al. Detection of SARS-CoV-2 genomic and subgenomic RNA in retina and optic nerve of patients with COVID-19. British Journal of Ophthalmology [Internet]. 2022;**106**(9):1313-1317. DOI: 10.1136/bjophthalmol-2020-318618

[17] Casagrande M, Fitzek A, Püschel K, Aleshcheva G, Schultheiss H-P, Berneking L, et al. Detection of SARS-CoV-2 in human retinal biopsies of deceased COVID-19 patients. Ocular Immunology and Inflammation [Internet]. 2020;**28**(5):721-725. DOI: 10.1080/09273948.2020.1770301

[18] Menuchin-Lasowski Y, Schreiber A, Lecanda A, Mecate-Zambrano A, Brunotte L, Psathaki OE, et al. SARS-CoV-2 infects and replicates in photoreceptor and retinal ganglion cells of human retinal organoids. Stem Cell Reports [Internet]. 2022;**17**(4):789-803. DOI: 10.1016/j.stemcr.2022.02.015

[19] Baig AM, Khaleeq A, Ali U, Syeda H. Evidence of the COVID-19 virus targeting the CNS: Tissue distribution, host–virus interaction, and proposed neurotropic mechanisms. ACS Chemical Neuroscience [Internet]. 2020;**11**(7):995-998. DOI: 10.1021/acschemneuro.0c00122

[20] Tang N, Li D, Wang X, Sun Z. Abnormal coagulation parameters are associated with poor prognosis in patients with novel coronavirus pneumonia. Journal of Thrombosis and Haemostasis [Internet]. 2020;**18**(4):844-847. DOI: 10.1111/jth.14768

[21] Alomari SO, Abou-Mrad Z, Bydon A. COVID-19 and the central nervous system. Clinical Neurology and Neurosurgery [Internet]. 2020;**198**(106116):106116. DOI: 10.1016/j.clineuro.2020.106116

[22] Sawalha K, Adeodokun S, Kamoga G-R. COVID-19-induced acute bilateral optic neuritis. Journal of Investigative Medicine High Impact Case Reports [Internet]. 2020;**8**. DOI: 10.1177/2324709620976018

[23] Zhou S, Jones-Lopez EC, Soneji DJ, Azevedo CJ, Patel VR. Myelin oligodendrocyte glycoprotein antibody–associated optic neuritis and myelitis in COVID-19. Journal of Neuro-Ophthalmology [Internet]. 2020;**40**(3):398-402. DOI: 10.1097/wno.0000000000001049

[24] Behera G, Gera P, Stephen M, Jose A, Thabah MM, Wadwekar V. Bilateral optic neuritis and facial palsy following COVID-19 infection. Cureus [Internet]. 2022;**14**(9):e28735. DOI: 10.7759/cureus.28735

[25] Dinkin M, Gao V, Kahan J, Bobker S, Simonetto M, Wechsler P, et al. COVID-19 presenting with ophthalmoparesis from cranial nerve palsy. Neurology [Internet]. 2020;**95**(5):221-223. DOI: 10.1212/wnl.0000000000009700

[26] Tonkal A, Alamri AA, AlMaghrabi SJ, Mozahim NF, Mozahim SF, Alsubaie SA,

et al. Cranial nerve impairment associated with COVID-19 infections: A systematic review. Cureus [Internet]. 2022;**14**(11):e31997. DOI: 10.7759/cureus.31997

[27] Gutiérrez-Ortiz C, Méndez-Guerrero A, Rodrigo-Rey S, San Pedro-Murillo E, Bermejo-Guerrero L, Gordo-Mañas R, et al. Miller fisher syndrome and polyneuritis cranialis in COVID-19. Neurology [Internet]. 2020;**95**(5):e601-e605. DOI: 10.1212/wnl.0000000000009619

[28] Mao L, Jin H, Wang M, Hu Y, Chen S, He Q, et al. Neurologic manifestations of hospitalized patients with coronavirus disease 2019 in Wuhan, China. JAMA Neurology [Internet]. 2020;**77**(6):683. DOI: 10.1001/jamaneurol.2020.1127

[29] Kharat A, Simon M, Guérin C. Prone position in COVID 19-associated acute respiratory failure. Current Opinion in Critical Care [Internet]. 2022;**28**(1):57-65. DOI: 10.1097/mcc.0000000000000900

[30] Fonollosa A, Hernández-Rodríguez J, Cuadros C, Giralt L, Sacristán C, Artaraz J, et al. Characterizing covid-19–related retinal vascular occlusions: A case series and review of the literature. Retina [Internet]. 2022;**42**(3):465-475. DOI: 10.1097/iae.0000000000003327

[31] Voicu S, Ketfi C, Stépanian A, Chousterman BG, Mohamedi N, Siguret V, et al. Pathophysiological processes underlying the high prevalence of deep vein thrombosis in critically ill COVID-19 patients. Frontiers in Physiology [Internet]. 2020;**11**:608788. DOI: 10.3389/fphys.2020.608788

[32] Klein R. The 15-year cumulative incidence of retinal vein occlusion: The beaver dam eye study. Archives of Ophthalmology [Internet]. 2008;**126**(4):513. DOI: 10.1001/archopht.126.4.513

[33] O'Mahoney PRA, Wong DT, Ray JG. Retinal vein occlusion and traditional risk factors for atherosclerosis. Archives of Ophthalmology [Internet]. 2008;**126**(5):692-699. DOI: 10.1001/archopht.126.5.692

[34] Sanjay S, Srinivasan P, Jayadev C, Mahendradas P, Gupta A, Kawali A, et al. Post COVID-19 ophthalmic manifestations in an Asian Indian male. Ocular Immunology and Inflammation [Internet]. 2021;**29**(4):656-661. DOI: 10.1080/09273948.2020.1870147

[35] Acharya S, Diamond M, Anwar S, Glaser A, Tyagi P. Unique case of central retinal artery occlusion secondary to COVID-19 disease. IDCases [Internet]. 2020;**21**(e00867):e00867. DOI: 10.1016/j.idcr.2020.e00867

[36] Costa ÍF, Bonifácio LP, Bellissimo-Rodrigues F, Rocha EM, Jorge R, Bollela VR, et al. Ocular findings among patients surviving COVID-19. Scientific Reports [Internet]. 2021;**11**(1):11085. DOI: 10.1038/s41598-021-90482-2

[37] Castro CS, Ferreira AS, Silva NP, Lume MR, Furtado MJ. Paracentral acute middle maculopathy after COVID-19 disease: Multimodal evaluation. Retinal Cases and Brief Reports [Internet]. 2022;**17**(6):791-796. DOI: 10.1097/icb.0000000000001301

[38] Virgo J, Mohamed M. Paracentral acute middle maculopathy and acute macular neuroretinopathy following SARS-CoV-2 infection. Eye [Internet]. 2020;**34**(12):2352-2353. DOI: 10.1038/s41433-020-1069-8

[39] Rahimy E, Kuehlewein L, Sadda SR, Sarraf D. Paracentral acute middle maculopathy: What we knew then and

what we know now. Retina [Internet]. 2015;**35**(10):1921-1930. DOI: 10.1097/IAE.0000000000000785

[40] Kalaw FGP, Warter A, Cavichini M, Knight D, Li A, Deussen D, et al. Retinal tissue and microvasculature loss in COVID-19 infection. Scientific Reports [Internet]. 2023;**13**(1):5100. DOI: 10.1038/s41598-023-31835-x

[41] Verdecchia P, Cavallini C, Spanevello A, Angeli F. COVID-19: ACE2centric infective disease? Hypertension [Internet]. 2020;**76**(2):294-299. DOI: 10.1161/HYPERTENSIONAHA.120.15353

[42] Teo KYC, Invernizzi A, Staurenghi G, Cheung CMG. COVID-19-related retinal micro-vasculopathy – A review of current evidence. American Journal of Ophthalmology [Internet]. 2022;**235**:98-110. DOI: 10.1016/j.ajo.2021.09.019

[43] Invernizzi A, Torre A, Parrulli S, Zicarelli F, Schiuma M, Colombo V, et al. Retinal findings in patients with COVID-19: Results from the SERPICO-19 study. EClinicalMedicine [Internet]. 2020;**27**(100550):100550. DOI: 10.1016/j.eclinm.2020.100550

[44] Kal M, Winiarczyk M, Zarębska-Michaluk D, Odrobina D, Cieśla E, Płatkowska-Adamska B, et al. Long-term effect of SARS-CoV-2 infection on the retinal and choroidal microvasculature. Journal of Clinical Medicine [Internet]. 2023;**12**(7):2528. DOI: 10.3390/jcm12072528

[45] Verdoni L, Mazza A, Gervasoni A, Martelli L, Ruggeri M, Ciuffreda M, et al. An outbreak of severe Kawasaki-like disease at the Italian epicentre of the SARS-CoV-2 epidemic: An observational cohort study. Lancet [Internet]. 2020;**395**(10239):1771-1778. DOI: 10.1016/s0140-6736(20)31103-x

[46] Becker RC. COVID-19 update: Covid-19-associated coagulopathy. Journal of Thrombosis and Thrombolysis [Internet]. 2020;**50**(1):54-67. DOI: 10.1007/s11239-020-02134-3

[47] Shulman ST, Rowley AH. Kawasaki disease: Insights into pathogenesis and approaches to treatment. Nature Reviews Rheumatology [Internet]. 2015;**11**(8):475-482. DOI: 10.1038/nrrheum.2015.54

[48] Esper F, Shapiro ED, Weibel C, Ferguson D, Landry ML, Kahn JS. Association between a novel human coronavirus and Kawasaki disease. The Journal of Infectious Diseases [Internet]. 2005;**191**(4):499-502. DOI: 10.1086/428291

[49] Quintana-Castanedo L, Feito-Rodríguez M, Fernández-Alcalde C, Granados-Fernández M, Montero-Vega D, Mayor-Ibarguren A, et al. Concurrent chilblains and retinal vasculitis in a child with COVID-19. Journal of the European Academy of Dermatology and Venereology [Internet]. 2020;**34**(12):e764-e766. DOI: 10.1111/jdv.16801

[50] Sanjay S, Agrawal S, Jayadev C, Kawali A, Gowda PB, Shetty R, et al. Posterior segment manifestations and imaging features post-COVID-19. Medical Hypothesis, Discovery & Innovation in Ophthalmology [Internet]. 2021;**10**(3):95-106. DOI: 10.51329/mehdiophthal1427

[51] Chan AX, Ritter M, Bakhoum MF. Bilateral cotton wool spots after ambulatory COVID-19. International Journal of Infectious Diseases [Internet]. 2021;**105**:414-415. DOI: 10.1016/j.ijid.2021.02.119

[52] Landecho MF, Yuste JR, Gándara E, Sunsundegui P, Quiroga J, Alcaide AB,

et al. COVID-19 retinal microangiopathy as an in vivo biomarker of systemic vascular disease? Journal of Internal Medicine [Internet]. 2021;**289**(1): 116-120. DOI: 10.1111/joim.13156

[53] Jaworski C. Morphology of the HIV versus the diabetic cotton wool spot. Optometry and Vision Science [Internet]. 2000;**77**(11):600-604. DOI: 10.1097/00006324-200011000-00010

[54] Akram MU, Akbar S, Hassan T, Khawaja SG, Yasin U, Basit I. Data on fundus images for vessels segmentation, detection of hypertensive retinopathy, diabetic retinopathy and papilledema. Data Brief [Internet]. 2020;**29**(105282):105282. DOI: 10.1016/j.dib.2020.105282

[55] Rai AS, Freund P, Margolin EA, Micieli JA. Numerous cotton wool spots from giant cell arteritis. Journal of Clinical Rheumatology [Internet]. 2020;**26**(5):e124. DOI: 10.1097/RHU.0000000000000995

[56] Pereira LA, Soares LCM, Nascimento PA, Cirillo LRN, Sakuma HT, Veiga GL da, et al. Retinal findings in hospitalised patients with severe COVID-19. British Journal of Ophthalmology [Internet]. 2022;106(1):102-105. DOI: 10.1136/bjophthalmol-2020-317576

[57] Zago Filho LA, Lima LH, Melo GB, Zett C, Farah ME. Vitritis and outer retinal abnormalities in a patient with COVID-19. Ocular Immunology and Inflammation [Internet]. 2020;**28**(8):1298-1300. DOI: 10.1080/09273948.2020.1821898

[58] Hepokur M, Gunes M, Durmus E, Aykut V, Esen F, Oguz H. Long-term follow-up of choroidal changes following COVID-19 infection: Analysis of choroidal thickness and choroidal vascularity index. Canadian Journal of Ophthalmology [Internet]. 2023;**58**(1):59-65. DOI: 10.1016/j.jcjo.2021.06.020

[59] Bayram N, Gundogan M, Ozsaygılı C, Adelman RA. Posterior ocular structural and vascular alterations in severe COVID-19 patients. Arbeitsphysiologie [Internet]. 2022;**260**(3):993-1004. DOI: 10.1007/s00417-021-05420-9

[60] Bariş Üçer M, Cevher S. How does Covid-19 affect the choroidal structures at the early post-infectious period? Journal Francais D Ophtalmologie [Internet]. 2023;**46**(2):106-113. DOI: 10.1016/j.jfo.2022.08.003

[61] Abdelmassih Y, Azar G, Bonnin S, Scemama Timsit C, Vasseur V, Spaide RF, et al. COVID-19 associated choroidopathy. Journal of Clinical Medicine [Internet]. 2021;**10**(20):4686. DOI: 10.3390/jcm10204686

Chapter 10

Managing COVID-19 Variants: Mapping Data from the International Clinical Trials Registry Platform

Duduzile Ndwandwe, Musawenkosi Ndlovu, Asanda Mayeye, Nomahlubi Luphondo, Ndivhuwo Muvhulawa, Yonela Ntamo, Phiwayinkosi V. Dludla and Charles Shey Wiysonge

Abstract

The COVID-19 pandemic has presented an ongoing global challenge, marked by the emergence of multiple SARS-CoV-2 variants. Effective management of these variants necessitates a comprehensive understanding of their clinical impact and the development of targeted interventions. This study explores the landscape of clinical trials giving a better understanding of the COVID-19 variants registered on the International Clinical Trials Registry Platform (ICTRP). Leveraging data from the ICTRP, we conducted an extensive mapping to assess basic characteristic features of registered clinical trials, while also giving an overview of currently used therapeutics, vaccines, and diagnostic tools specifically tailored to combat SARS-CoV-2 variants. Our analysis also provides valuable insights into the geographical distribution, trial design, and therapeutic modalities targeted at these variants. By synthesizing and visualizing this data, we aim to facilitate global collaboration, resource allocation, and evidence-based decision-making in the ongoing fight against COVID-19 variants. This chapter underscores the significance of the ITCRP registry for understanding the evolving pandemic landscape and highlights the ongoing efforts to confront the challenges posed by SARS-CoV-2 variants. The chapter also highlights essential considerations relevant to the management of COVID-19 variants in low- and middle-income countries with limited health infrastructure.

Keywords: COVID-19 pandemic, SARS-CoV-2 variants, clinical impact, targeted interventions, clinical trials

1. Introduction

The global COVID-19 pandemic began in late 2019, where it suddenly propelled the scientific community to come up with solutions to unravel the mysteries of the SARS-CoV-2 virus [1]. Until this day, the COVID-19 pandemic continues to challenge humanity in unprecedented ways, driving a need to develop effective vaccines and treatments to combat the virus [2, 3]. The prime example is the redefining feature of long COVID, which occurs more often in people who had severe COVID-19 illness [4]. In fact, it has become essential to understand the dynamic nature of SARS-CoV-2 variants as part of an ongoing battle against this virus. This includes exploring the genetic changes that underpin the ever-evolving world of SARS-CoV-2 variants, potentially contributing to the course of the pandemic [1].

The COVID-19 pandemic has witnessed the emergence of several distinct SARS-CoV-2 variants, each characterized by unique genetic mutations [5]. Some of the most notable variants include the Alpha variant (B.1.1.7), initially identified in the United Kingdom, and known for its significantly rapid infectious rate [6]. This variant quickly spread to numerous countries, leading to concerns about its potential to drive surges in cases [6]. Following closely behind was the Beta variant (B.1.351), first discovered in South Africa [7]. This variant raised considerable alarm within the scientific community due to mutations in the spike protein that appeared to reduce the effectiveness of certain vaccines [5, 7]. The Gamma variant (P.1), also originating in Brazil, shared genetic similarities with the Beta variant [8]. Researchers noted that both variants had mutations in common, particularly within the spike protein. In late 2021, the Delta variant (B.1.617.2) emerged as a dominant force among the COVID-19 variants [8, 9]. Originating in India, Delta exhibited unprecedented transmissibility, leading to rapid and widespread infections. By now high-quality sequences of Delta (B.1.617.2) and Delta Plus (AY.1 or B.1.617.2.1) variants have been used to uncover the prevalence of mutations in the entire SARS-CoV-2 genome [10]. Lastly, the Omicron variant (B.1.1.529) surfaced, characterized by an unusually high number of genetic mutations, particularly in the spike protein [11]. Omicron's emergence raised concerns about its potential to evade immunity generated by previous infections or vaccinations [11]. The appearance of Omicron underscored the need for ongoing vigilance and adaptability in the fight against COVID-19 and its evolving variants, especially during the fourth wave of the pandemic [5, 12].

The past few years have seen extensive research being undertaken to understand their behavior, impact on disease severity, vaccine resistance potential, as well as relevant implications for diagnostics and treatments [5, 8, 12]. Thus, it become important to monitor and study these variants as part of the ongoing efforts to combat the evolving COVID-19 pandemic. While much work has focused on the short-term effects of COVID-19 variants, a significant research gap lies in comprehending the long-term consequences of variant exposure on immunity [13–16]. These studies have shown that different variants exhibit varying degrees of immune escape, potentially impacting the effectiveness of vaccines and natural immunity [13–16]. However, there is limited data on how these variants may influence the duration and strength of immunity against subsequent infections or the longevity of vaccine-induced protection. Thus, there is a need to continuously reinforce efforts our understanding the durability of immunity in individuals exposed to different variants, including reinfection rates, and vaccine breakthrough cases remains crucial for informing vaccination strategies, booster campaigns, and long-term pandemic management [17–23]. This will surely enhance the capacity ability to adapt our public health measures and vaccination approaches effectively as the virus continues to evolve.

This chapter seeks to contribute to the collective knowledge to effectively monitoring the evolution of viral variants and their potential impact on public health. The International Clinical Trials Registry Platform (ICTRP) holds immense significance in the field of medical research and healthcare. It serves as a global repository for clinical trial registrations, fostering transparency, accountability, and accessibility of crucial research endeavors [24]. By providing a centralized platform for researchers to register their trials, ICTRP ensures that valuable data on clinical trials are publicly available, enabling fellow scientists, healthcare professionals, and policymakers to access comprehensive information. This transparency not only promotes ethical research practices but also facilitates collaboration and the sharing of critical findings, eventually advancing medical knowledge and improving patient care worldwide [24]. In the context of public health crises like the COVID-19 pandemic, ICTRP's role in disseminating vital trial information is even more pronounced, allowing for informed decision-making and the rapid development of life-saving interventions. In this cross-sectional survey of the ICTRP database, we report on the trends in the clinical trials registered on COVID-19 variants, including relevant data on clinical trials reporting on the Alpha, Beta, Delta, Gamma, and Omicron variants. The chapter also highlights essential considerations relevant to the management of COVID-19 variants in low- and middle-income countries with limited health infrastructure.

2. Methodology

2.1 Source and data description

This was a comprehensive analysis of the trends in clinical trials registered with the ICTRP (https://www.who.int/clinical-trials-registry-platform) [24]. This platform collects clinical data from registries across the globe, in the process becoming a one-stop portal to access clinical trial records. The study employed the World Health Organization (WHO) classification of a clinical trial: 'any research study that prospectively assigns human participants or groups of humans to one or more health-related interventions to evaluate the effects on health outcomes' [25, 26]. An advanced search function of ICTRP was used to identify relevant clinical trials, registered on 20 August 2023.

2.2 An approach for data analysis and management

An independent researcher (M.N.) made use of the world WHO-ICTRP portal to download relevant data on the 20th of August 2023. During this process, data was exported into an Excel spreadsheet before other researchers (N.M. and P.V.D.) performed quality checks. For each record, some of the critical data items collected included the trial registry source, date of registration, recruitment status, retrospective flag, gender, trial phases, and intervention model. Additional information collected were the biomarkers, symptoms, recovery time, imaging findings, viral load, immune response, psychology, and other measures corresponding to each COVID-19 variant. Collected data items allowed for a comprehensive analysis of trends and patterns across COVID-19 variants within an Excel spreadsheet.

3. Characteristics for included clinical trials

3.1 Study selection

This section reports on clinical trials conducted on the five COVID-19 variants, including the Alpha, Beta, Delta, Gamma, and Omicron. Data was retrieved per

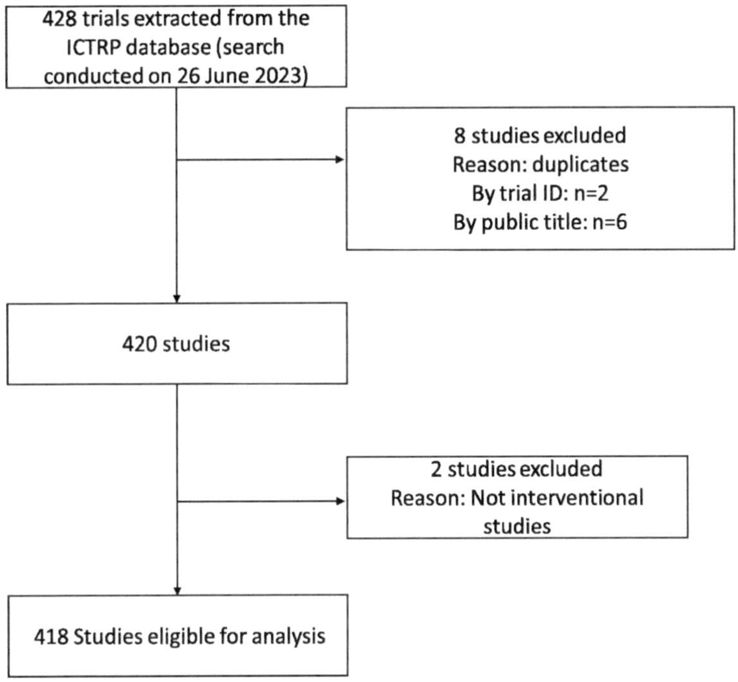

Figure 1.
Flowchart illustrating the process of clinical trials (n = 418) on the five COVID-19 variants, including the alpha, Beta, Delta, gamma, and omicron. Data was retrieved per individual variant from the international clinical trials registry platform on the 20th of august 2023.

individual variant from the WHO-ICTRP. Initially, the dataset included 428 studies. However, a total of 8 duplicated studies were removed, of those, 2 were eliminated due to sharing the same trial ID, while 6 were excluded for having identical titles. Additionally, 2 studies were removed as they did not meet the inclusion criteria or did not give sufficient information on COVID-19 variants. Overall, 10 studies were eliminated, leaving a total of 418 studies for further analysis (**Figure 1**). These 418 studies have been registered since 1999 to 2023 (**Figure 1**). During the year 1999 to 2004, there were very few studies registered. The lowest being in 2001 with no registered studies. Notably, the most significant changes occurred after 2020, where the highest reported studies were seen between 2021 and 2022.

3.2 Data on the diverse clinical trial registry sources

The WHO clearly states that access to the ICTRP is necessary to safeguard a complete view of research to those involved in healthcare decision making [27]. This will surely improve research transparency and will eventually reinforce the validity and value of the scientific evidence base [27]. The ICTRP registry pools together or gives access to data from different clinical trial registries. In terms of the COIVD-19 variants, the combined data pooled from the clinical trials shows that the Alpha (n = 104) variant had the highest number of records, followed by Beta (n = 93), Delta (n = 37), Gamma (n = 68), and Omicron (n = 116) (**Table 1**). The ClinicalTrials.gov remains the predominant source of accessing data for clinical trials on COVID-19 variants, including the Alpha, Beta, Delta, Gamma, and Omicron (**Table 1**). The next registry is the Iranian Registry of Clinical Trials (IRCT), followed by the Clinical Trials Registry- India

Trial characteristic	Variants				
	Alpha(*n* = **104**), *n* (%)	**Beta**(*n* = **93**) *n* (%)	**Delta**(*n* = **37**) *n* (%)	**Gamma**(*n* = **68**) *n* (%)	**Omicron**(**n** = **116**) *n* (%)
Trial registry source					
ANZCTR	8, (7.69)	N/A	1, (2.70)	3, (4.41)	2, (1.72)
ChiCTR	11, (10.58)	1, (1.08)	6, (16.22)	N/A	36, (31.03)
ClinicalTrials gov	28, (26.92)	39, (41.93)	18, (48.65)	21, (30.88)	56, (48.28)
CTRI	12, (11.53)	5, (5.38)	2, (5.41)	14, (20.59)	5, (4.31)
DRKS	3, (2.88)	1, (1.08)	N/A	6, (8.82)	1, (0.86)
ISRCTN	9, (8.65)	4, (4.30)	1, (2.70)	4, (5.88)	3, (2.59)
PACTR	1, (0.96)	1, (1.08)	1, (2.70)	N/A	1, (0.86)
TCTR	1, (0.96)	1, (1.08)	3, (8.11)	N/A	2, (1.72)
IRCT	16, (15.38)	29, (31.18)	N/A	7, (10.29)	1, (0.86)
RPCEC	6, (5.77)	N/A	N/A	N/A	1, (0.86)
ITMCTR	N/A	N/A	4, (10.81)	N/A	8, (6.90)
REPEC	N/A	1, (1.08)	N/A	N/A	N/A
SLCTR	1, (0.96)	N/A	N/A	N/A	N/A
EU-CTR	5, (4.81)	9, (9.68)	1, (2.70)	8, (11.76)	N/A
JPRN	N/A	1, (1.08)	N/A	1, (1.47)	N/A
REBEC	2, (1.92)	N/A	N/A	N/A	N/A
LTR	N/A	N/A	N/A	3, (4.41)	N/A
Date of registration					
2019	N/A	N/A	N/A	1, (1.47)	N/A
2020	60, (57.69)	56, (60.22)	1, (2.70)	25, (36.76)	1, (0.86)
2021	24, (23.08)	17, (18.28)	13, (35.14)	24, (35.29)	2, (1.72)
2022	16, (15, 38)	18, (19.35)	20, (54.05)	15, (22.06)	88, (75.86)
2023	4, (3.85)	2, (2.15)	3, (8.11)	3, (4.41)	25, (21.55)
Recruitment status					
Recruiting	34, (32.69)	32, (34.41)	13, (35.14)	22, (32.35)	48, (41.38)
Not recruiting	68, (65.38)	55, (59.14)	23, (62.16)	39, (57.35)	67, (57.76)
Authorized	2, (1.92)	N/A	N/A	7, (10.29)	N/A
Not specified	N/A	6, (6.45)	1, (2.70)	N/A	1, (0.86)
Retrospective flag					
Yes	76, (73.08)	64, (68.82)	25, (67.57)	52, (76.47)	84, (72.41)
No	28, (26.92)	29, (31.13)	12, (32.43)	16, (23.53)	32, (27.59)
Gender					
Both gender	86, (82.69)	82, (92.47)	35, (94.59)	52, (76.47)	111, (95.69)
Female	1, (0.96)	1, (1.08)	N/A	1, (1.47)	N/A
Male	1, (0.96)	N/A	N/A	N/A	N/A
Not specified	N/A	6, (6.45)	2, (5.41)	15, (22.06)	5, (4.31)
Trial phases					

Trial characteristic	Variants				
	Alpha(n = **104**), n (%)	**Beta**(n = **93**) n (%)	**Delta**(n = **37**) n (%)	**Gamma**(n = **68**) n (%)	**Omicron**(**n** = **116**) n (%)
Phase I	6, (5.77)	4, (4.17)	N/A	5, (7.81)	8, (6.90)
Phase II	24, (23.08)	24, (25)	11, (29, 80)	11, (17.19)	14, (12.07)
Phase III	19, (18, 27)	36, (37.5)	7, (18.92)	11, (17.19)	15, (12.93)
Phase IV	10, (9.62)	5, (5.21	N/A	3, (4.69)	6, (5.17)
Phase I-II	5, (4.81)	1, (1.04)	N/A	1, (56)	2, (1.72)
Phase II-III	5, (4.81)	9, (9.38)	N/A	2, (3.13)	4, (3.45)
Phase III-IV	1, (0.96)	N/A	N/A	N/A	1, (0.86)
Not applicable	24, (23.08)	12, (12.50)	N/A	17, (26, 56)	31, (26.72)
Intervention Model					
Cross-over assignment	5, (4.81)	9, (9.67)	1, (2.70)	2, (2.94)	2, (3)
Factorial assignment	1, (0.96)	1, (1.08)	1, (2.70)	N/A	1, (1)
Parallel assignment	65, (62.5)	74, (79.57)	22, (59.46)	38, (55.88)	54, (76)
Sequential assignment	1, (0.96)	2, (2.15)	1, (2.70)	1, (1.47)	2, (3)
Single group assignment	4, (3.85)	1, (1.08)	1, (2.70)	1, (1.47)	4, (5)
Other	2, (1.92)	3, (3.22)	5, (13.51)	15, (22.06)	4, (6)
None (open labeled)	20, (19.23)	3, (3.22)	6, (16.22)	1, (1.47	4, (6)

ChiCTR, Chinese Clinical Trial Registry; CTRI, Clinical Trials Registry-India; IRCT, Iranian Registry of Clinical Trials; ISRCTN, International Standard Randomized Controlled Trial Number; ITMCTR, International Traditional Medicine Clinical Trial Registry; TCTR, Thai Clinical Trials Registry, RPCEC, Cuban Public Registry of Clinical Trials; PACTR, Pan African Clinical Trials Registry; ANZCTR, Australian New Zealand Clinical Trials Registry; DRKS, German Clinical Trials Register; SLCTR, Sri Lanka Clinical Trials Registry, REPEC, The Peruvian Clinical Trials Registry; LTR, Dutch Trial Registry. CAM- Complementary and Alternative Medicine.

Table 1.
Characteristics of the clinical trials registered for the five COVID-19 variants (alpha, Beta, Delta, gamma, and omicron).

(CTRI), International Standard Randomized Controlled Trial Number (ISRCTN), EU Clinical Trials Register, Chinese Clinical Trial Registry (ChiCTR), Australian New Zealand Clinical Trials Registry (ANZCTR), and German Clinical Trials Register (DRKS), respectively (**Table 1**). However, very limited data and even records are missing for the other clinical trial registries, including the Pan-African Clinical Trials Registry (PANCTR), Thai Clinical Trials Registry (TCTR), and others (**Table 1**).

3.3 Data on the clinical trial registration and recruitment status

Table 1 results also showed a year-dependent registration of clinical trials on different COVID-19 variants, starting from 2019 to 2023. As expected, before the first outbreak was reported towards the end of 2019 [28], limited or no information was available on the recorded clinical trials on all COVID-19 variants (**Table 1**). In fact, it was only in 2020 that much of the clinical trials were recorded for both the Alpha (n = 60), and Beta (n = 56) variants, because they were the first variants to emerge. The years 2021 to 2022 recorded a steady registration of clinical trials across all COVID-19 variants (**Table 1**). However, more clinical trials were registered for the Omicron variant (75%) by the year 2022 (**Table 1**) since it first emerged and became the most transmissible variant towards the end of 2022 [29]. By the year 2023, the registered trials fell significantly across the years, although the Omicron (21%) variant still showed a higher number of registered clinical trials compared to the Alpha (3%), Beta (2%), and Delta (8%) (**Table 1**). There was a decline in trial recruitment status for all COVID-19 variants, based on the progressing years, especially lower for the years 2023 (**Table 1**).

3.4 Data on the gender and type of clinical trial

Table 1 also gives information on the gender of participants included within these clinical trials and was evenly distributed across both males and females. Only a few clinical trials included males or females only. In terms of trial phases, most records showed predominant allocation to phase II and phase III, across all COVID-19 variants (**Table 1**). Meaning these clinical trials were likely to be conducted to uncover the safety and efficacy of interventions or vaccines [30]. Interestingly, it was also apparent that a few records did not specify the type of phase of other clinical trial, including the Alpha (23%), Beta (12%), Gamma (26%), and the Omicron (26%) variants (**Table 1**). Moreover, for each category, retrospective flag scored above 60% for the Alpha, Beta, and the Omicron variants (**Table 1**).

3.5 Data on different interventions for COVID-19 variants

Table 2 also gives information on the different interventions or approaches that have been used for each of the COVID-19 variants, including pharmacotherapy, vaccine therapy, complementary and alternative medicine, and educational therapy. Other interventions included diagnostic (devices), behavior, and dietary supplements. The intervention model was mostly parallel across all COVID-19 variants (**Table 2**), where the clinical study likely involved two or more groups of participants receiving different interventions [31]. Indeed, more than 50% of clinical trials registered for the Alpha, Beta, and Gamma variants focused on pharmacotherapy intervention either as mono or combination therapy (**Table 2**). The most common agents studied in the registered clinical trials include Lopinavir/Ritonavir, Dexamethasone, and Ribavirin. Vaccine therapy was also among the most studied interventions, for the Alpha (19%), Beta (19%), Delta (22%), Gamma (15%), and Omicron (45%) variants (**Table 2**). Notably, Sinocelltech (SCTV01 E&C), mRNA 1273, Comirnaty, and BNT162b2 were among the most common vaccines used for the registered trials. The complementary and alternative medicine investigated against the five COVID-19 encompasses mostly Chinese medicine such as Ayurveda and Lianhua Qingwen (**Table 2**). Other interventions, including those simply educational scored less in terms of clinical trials registry (**Table 2**).

Intervention type	Example	Alpha (%)	Beta (%)	Delta (%)	Gamma (%)	Omicron (%)
Pharmacotherapy	Lopinavir/ Ritonavir, Remsdivir, Interferon beta-1α, Interferon beta-1β, IFN-G, Mozobil, Paxlovid, Ribavirin, Dexamethasone, Anakinra	54, (51.92)	60, (64.52)	2, (5.41)	38, (55.88)	6, (6.12)
CAM	Ayuderva, Herbal medicine*, Lianhua Qingwen, JieJiXuanFeiChuYi Granule	4, (3.84)	4, (4.30)	6, (16.22)	N/A	15, (15.31)
Vaccine therapy	SCTV01E &C, mRNA-1273, BNT162b2, Comirnaty, Sinopharm, RBD-based ARVAC-CG, NVX-CoV2373	19, (18.27)	19, (20.43)	22, (59.46)	15, (22.06)	45, (45.92)
Education	Yoga modules, Mental health knowledge, psychological lessons.	4, (3.84)	1, (1.08))	N/A	N/A	N/A
Others	Dietary supplements, Diagnostic, Behavioral, Nitric oxide gas	16, (15.09)	9, (6.68)	2, (5.41)	15, (22.06)	12, (12.24)
None		N/A	N/A	5, (13.51)	N/A	20, (20.41)

**Different herbs; mRNA vaccine (mRNA-1273), Sinocelltech (SCTV01), Interferon beta-1α (SNG001), Complementary and alternative medicine (CAM), Interferon-gamma human recombinant (IFN-G), NVX-CoV-Novavax COVID-19 (NVX-CoV2373).*

Table 2.
An overview of interventions corresponding to different types of intervention for each COVID-19 variant.

4. Data on the different primary outcomes corresponding to each COVID-19 variant

The devastating impact of the different COVID-19 variants on public health and control measures underlines the need for continued vigilance and adherence to preventive measures such as mask-wearing, physical distancing, and vaccination. Additionally, ongoing research has focused on evaluating the efficacy of existing treatments, including vaccines for their targeted impact to mitigate the associated complications. The response to the interventions made in the registered trials was measured by the evaluation of some common primary outcomes. In **Table 2**, the primary outcomes are categorized into different groups, including biomarkers, COVID-19 symptoms, respiration rate, recovery time, image findings, viral load, geometric mean titers, and psychological effects. Notably, the most common biomarkers included measuring several pro-inflammatory markers like interleukins, lymphocytes, tumor necrosis factor-alpha (TNF-α), C-reactive protein (CRP), and cytokines, as well as glucose-related markers and insulin (**Table 3**). These biomarkers were regularly recorded for all COVID-19 variants. In terms of symptoms, optimal physical strength

Primary outcome	Alpha	Beta	Delta	Gamma	Omicron
Biomarkers	CRP, PAI-1, TNF-α, IFN-α, cytokines, creatinine	HAS, IFN- β, CRP, insulin, IL-6, siderophin, C-peptides	Interleukins, IFN-(α, β, γ), T lymphocytes, IgG	CRP, interleukins, D dimer, Ferritin, lymphocytes, IFN- γ	CRP, serum cytokines, blood sugar, T lymphocytes, IgG,
Symptoms	Vital signs	Cough, fever, headache, Body temperature	Physical activity, sleep	Fatigue, muscle strength, weakness, nausea	Clinical symptom score, taste, social stigma, sleep, fever, sore throat, fatigue, headache, pain, cough, Body temp, Insomnia, diarrhea
Respiration rate	VFD, OS	OS, RC, OR	N/A	VFD	VFD
Recovery time	NA	Hospitalization period	N/A	N/A	Hospitalization length, CBV, VNCT, disease-free time,
Imaging findings	CT-scans	CT-scans	NA	CT scan	Chest CT scan, MMSE, Image metrics
Viral load	qPCR (CVL)	qPCR (CVL)	qPCR (CVL)	N/A	CT value (qPCR)
Immune response	GMT, NAb	GMT, NAb, COVID-19 antibodies	GMT, NAb	GMT, NAb	GMT, NaT, NAb
Psychology	N/A	N/A	Social stigma	Anxiety, Depression	SRAS, PSQI, Anxiety disorder scale 7,
Other measures	N/A	N/A	Nucleic acid tests, TCM syndrome score, Blood routine	N/A	Nucleic acid test, CiTAS-Chemotherapy-induced Taste Alteration, Pulmonary function test

VFD-Ventilation-free days, OS- Oxygen saturation, HSA-Human Serum albumin, CRP-C-reactive protein, PAI-1 – Plasminogen activator inhibitor-1; QPCR-quantitative polymerase chain reaction, RC-Respiratory capacity, OR-Oxygen requirement, IL-6- interleukin 6, NaT-Neutralizing Antibody Titers; CBV- Change from baseline vaccination, IgG-Immunoglobulin, VNCT-Virus negative conversion time, MMSE-Mini- Mental State Examination, SRAS-Self-Rating Anxiety Scale, PSQI-Pittsburgh Sleep Quality Index, GMT -Geometric mean titers, CVL-Change of Viral Load.

Table 3.
Primary outcomes corresponding to different types of intervention for each COVID-19 variant.

appeared to be predominantly assessed, including cough, fever, headache, body temperature, and fatigue across all COVID-19 variants (**Table 3**). However, even more clinical symptoms could be identified, including clinical symptom score, taste, social stigma, sleep, fever, sore throat, fatigue, headache, pain, cough, body temp, insomnia, and diarrhea (**Table 3**). Immune response appears to be one of the critical outcomes post-vaccinations, measured as geometric mean titer and determination of neutralizing antibody titers. Some trials for the Delta, Gamma, and Omicron variants studied the psychological response of individuals post-intervention, monitoring depression, social stigma, and anxiety (**Table 3**).

5. Discussion

In this chapter, we examine clinical data on the ever-evolving landscape of the COVID-19 pandemic, where new variants have emerged, presenting fresh challenges to our understanding and response. The comprehensive analysis of diverse clinical trial registry sources, as highlighted in this study, underscores the crucial role of the International ICTRP in healthcare decision-making and research transparency. The registration patterns revealed that as COVID-19 variants emerged, research efforts intensified, with the Alpha and Beta variants initially garnering significant attention due to their early appearance. In contrast, the Omicron variant, with its remarkable transmissibility, attracted a surge of clinical trials, reflecting the urgency in understanding and combating this new threat. Moreover, the study provides insights into the gender distribution of participants and the phases of clinical trials conducted for various COVID-19 variants. The balanced inclusion of both males and females in trials is noteworthy, contributing to more representative findings. Most clinical trials focused on phases II and III, indicating a primary focus on the safety and efficacy of the assessed interventions.

Moreover, the study sheds light on the diverse interventions employed to address COVID-19 variants, encompassing pharmacotherapy, vaccine therapy, complementary and alternative medicine, and to a lesser extent, the educational approaches. This multifaceted intervention landscape underscores the global effort to explore various strategies to combat the pandemic [32]. Notably, the vaccine therapy garnered significant attention across variants, emphasizing the central role of vaccination in pandemic management [33]. Overall, this comprehensive examination of clinical trial registry data highlights the impact of diverse COVID-19 variants on public health and a need to establish effective control measures or preventive strategies. Literature has increasingly covered these strategies, including mask-wearing, physical distancing, and vaccination, especially their instrumental role in mitigating the spread of the virus and preventing severe outcomes [34–36]. Indeed, as the pandemic continues to evolve, research efforts have continually assessed the effectiveness of existing treatments and interventions, with a particular focus on vaccines designed to target specific variants [37].

The evaluation of interventions within the registered clinical trials has been guided by various primary outcomes, categorized into distinct groups. Biomarkers have played a crucial role in determining immune response, with an emphasis on pro-inflammatory markers, interleukins, lymphocytes, TNF-α, C-reactive protein, and cytokines, which are likely to determine the severity of COVID-19 [12, 38]. In fact, the assessed biomarkers like blood glucose levels and insulins also indicate the surveillance of relevant risk of COVID-19 in patients with diabetes mellitus [39]. Interestingly, these biomarkers have been consistently assessed across trials for all COVID-19 variants, reflecting their importance in understanding the immune response and disease progression [40–42]. Moreover, primary outcomes related to COVID-19 have been a focal point of evaluation, with a particular emphasis on assessing optimal physical strength, including clinical symptoms such as cough, fever, headache, body temperature, and fatigue. However, a wide range of clinical symptoms has been monitored, encompassing clinical symptom scores, taste, social stigma, sleep patterns, sore throat, insomnia, diarrhea, and more. This comprehensive approach to symptom assessment reflects the complex nature of COVID-19's impact on individuals, especially in response to different COVID-19 variants [43–45].

Consistently highlighted within this chapter, is the critical role of monitoring the immune response, especially in the context of vaccinations. Evaluation has included measures such as geometric mean titers and the determination of neutralizing antibody titers, providing insights into the effectiveness of vaccines against different variants. Additionally, the psychological response of individuals post-intervention has been examined in some trials for variants like Delta, Gamma, and Omicron, with a focus on monitoring depression, social stigma, and anxiety. This holistic approach to outcome assessment is essential in comprehensively understanding the impact of interventions and treatments on individuals' physical and mental well-being.

6. Summary

In summary, this chapter provides a comprehensive exploration of the ever-evolving landscape of the COVID-19 pandemic, characterized by the emergence of diverse variants that pose ongoing challenges to our understanding and response. It highlights the pivotal role of the International ICTRP in promoting healthcare decision-making and research transparency, especially as research efforts intensified in response to new variants like Alpha, Beta, and Omicron. The study emphasizes the significance of balanced gender representation in clinical trials and the predominant focus on phases II and III, reflecting a primary concern for assessing intervention safety and efficacy. Additionally, the chapter discusses the wide array of interventions employed to combat COVID-19 variants, with vaccination as a central strategy. The evaluation of interventions within clinical trials encompasses various primary outcomes, including biomarkers crucial in assessing the severity of COVID-19.

7. Conclusions

In essence, this chapter highlights ongoing research, especially from clinical trial registries, informing on the importance of assessing the effectiveness of existing treatments and interventions, particularly vaccines targeting specific variants. This in-depth analysis of clinical trial registry data significantly contributes to our evolving understanding of COVID-19 and guides evidence-based strategies for combatting the pandemic and its myriad variants.

8. Future considerations, especially for poor health infrastructure in low-and-middle-income countries

The emergence of new variants of SARS-CoV-2 raises particular concerns for low- and middle-income countries (LMICs) with limited health infrastructure. These countries often face challenges in terms of healthcare resources, testing capacity, and access to vaccines, which can further exacerbate the impact of new variants on their populations.

1. Increased strain on healthcare systems: The introduction of more transmissible variants can lead to a surge in COVID-19 cases, placing a significant burden on healthcare systems that are already stretched thin. LMICs may struggle to cope with the increased demand for hospital beds, oxygen supply, and medical staff, resulting in compromised care for both COVID-19 patients and those requiring other healthcare services.

2. Limited testing and surveillance capabilities: Rapid and widespread testing is crucial for early detection and containment of new variants. However, LMICs often face challenges in terms of limited testing capacities and access to advanced genomic sequencing technologies. This can hinder their ability to monitor the emergence and spread of new variants, potentially delaying necessary public health responses.

3. Vaccine inequity and limited coverage: Vaccination campaigns play a critical role in mitigating the impact of new variants. However, many LMICs face challenges in accessing and distributing vaccines due to supply shortages, logistical hurdles, and vaccine inequity. Limited vaccine coverage in these countries can leave populations vulnerable to new variants, with potential implications for disease severity and mortality rates.

4. Inequitable access to therapeutics and treatments: The emergence of new variants may require the development and distribution of targeted therapeutics or treatments. However, LMICs may face challenges in accessing and affording these interventions, leading to disparities in healthcare access and outcomes.

5. Long-term socioeconomic impact: The ongoing impact of new variants can have long-term socioeconomic consequences for LMICs. The disruption of essential services, such as education, employment, and commerce, can deepen existing inequalities and hinder economic recovery efforts, further straining already fragile health systems.

Addressing these challenges requires international collaboration and support to strengthen health infrastructure in LMICs. This includes increasing testing capacities, enhancing genomic surveillance, ensuring equitable access to vaccines and therapeutics, and providing financial and technical assistance to bolster healthcare systems. It is crucial to prioritize the needs of LMICs and ensure that they have the resources and support necessary to effectively respond to the evolving threat posed by new variants.

Author contribution

All authors, including Musawenkosi Ndlovu, Asanda Mayeye, Nomahlubi Luphondo, Ndivhuwo Muvhulawa, Yonela Ntamo, Phiwayinkosi V. Dludla, and Charles Shey Wiysonge - wrote the manuscript, edited the revised draft, and approved the final version.

Funding statement

This work was supported in part by baseline funding from the South African Medical Research Council (SAMRC). The content hereof is the sole responsibility of the authors and do not necessarily represent the official views of the SAMRC or the funders.

Conflict of interest

The authors declare no conflict of interest.

Consent for publication

Not applicable. No individual person's data has been included in this manuscript.

Ethics approval

This is a review of already published studies and thus it does not require ethical approval.

Data availability and material

Data related to search strategy, study selection, and extraction items will be made available upon request after the manuscript is published.

Patient and public involvement

Patients and/or the public were not involved in the design, or conduct, or reporting, or dissemination plans of this research.

Abbreviations

ANZCTR	Australian New Zealand clinical trials registry
CAM	complementary and alternative medicine
CBV	change from baseline vaccination
ChiCTR	Chinese clinical trial registry
CRP-C	reactive protein
CTRI	clinical trials registry-India
CVL	change of viral load
DRKS	German clinical trials register
EU-CTR	EU clinical trials register
GMT	geometric mean titers

HAS	human serum albumin
ICTRP	international clinical trials registry platform
IFN	interferon
IgG	immunoglobulin
IL-6	interleukin 6
IRCT	Iranian registry of clinical trials
ISRCTN	international standard randomized controlled trial number
ITMCTR	international traditional medicine clinical trial registry
JPRN	Japan primary registries network
LMICs	low- and middle-income countries
LTR	Dutch trial registry
MMSE	mini- mental state examination
NaT	neutralizing antibody titers
OR	oxygen requirement
OS	oxygen saturation
PACTR	pan African clinical trials registry
PAI-1	plasminogen activator inhibitor-1
PSQI	Pittsburgh sleep quality index
QPCR	quantitative polymerase chain reaction
RC	respiratory capacity
ReBec	Brazilian clinical trials registry
REPEC	the Peruvian clinical trials registry
RPCEC	Cuban public registry of clinical trials
SARS-CoV-2	severe acute respiratory syndrome coronavirus 2
SLCTR	Sri Lanka clinical trials registry
SRAS	self-rating anxiety scale
TCTR	Thai clinical trials registry
TNF-α	factor-alpha
VFD	ventilation-free days
VNCT	virus negative conversion time
WHO	world health organization

Author details

Duduzile Ndwandwe[1*], Musawenkosi Ndlovu[1], Asanda Mayeye[1], Nomahlubi Luphondo[1], Ndivhuwo Muvhulawa[1,2], Yonela Ntamo[1], Phiwayinkosi V. Dludla[1,3] and Charles Shey Wiysonge[4]

1 Cochrane South Africa, South African Medical Research Council, Cape Town, South Africa

2 Department of Biochemistry, North-West University, Mafikeng Campus, South Africa

3 Department of Biochemistry and Microbiology, University of Zululand, Richards Bay, South Africa

4 World Health Organization Regional Office for Africa, Brazzaville, Republic of Congo

*Address all correspondence to: duduzile.ndwandwe@mrc.ac.za

References

[1] World Health Organization. Historical Working Definitions and Primary Actions for SARS-CoV-2 Variants. World Health Organization; 2023. Available from: https://www.who.int/publications/m/item/historical-working-definitions-and-primary-actions-for-sars-cov-2-variants [Accessed: September 1, 2023]

[2] Siddique A, Shahzad A, Lawler J, Mahmoud KA, Lee DS, Ali N, et al. Unprecedented environmental and energy impacts and challenges of COVID-19 pandemic. Environmental Research. 2021;**193**:110443

[3] Rutjes SA, Vennis IM, Wagner E, Maisaia V, Peintner L. Biosafety and biosecurity challenges during the COVID-19 pandemic and beyond. Frontiers in Bioengineering and Biotechnology. 2023;**11**:1117316

[4] Prevention CfDCa. Long COVID or Post-COVID Conditions. Prevention CfDCa. Available from: https://www.cdc.gov/coronavirus/2019-ncov/long-term-effects/index.html; [Accessed: September 2, 2023]

[5] Lippi G, Sanchis-Gomar F, Henry BM. COVID-19 and its long-term sequelae: What do we know in 2023? Polish Archives of Internal Medicine. 2023;**133**(4):16402

[6] Fiolet T, Kherabi Y, Mac Donald CJ, Ghosn J, Peiffer-Smadja N. Comparing COVID-19 vaccines for their characteristics, efficacy and effectiveness against SARS-CoV-2 and variants of concern: A narrative review. Clinical Microbiology and Infection. 2022;**28**(2):202-221

[7] Pavot V, Berry C, Kishko M, Anosova NG, Li L, Tibbitts T, et al. Beta variant COVID-19 protein booster vaccine elicits durable cross-neutralization against SARS-CoV-2 variants in non-human primates. Nature Communications. 2023;**14**(1):1309

[8] Pasquevich KA, Coria LM, Ceballos A, Mazzitelli B, Rodriguez JM, Demaría A, et al. Safety and immunogenicity of a SARS-CoV-2 gamma variant RBD-based protein adjuvanted vaccine used as booster in healthy adults. Nature Communications. 2023;**14**(1):4551

[9] Manjunath R, Gaonkar SL, Saleh EAM, Husain K. A comprehensive review on Covid-19 omicron (B.1.1.529) variant. Saudi Journal of Biological Sciences. 2022;**29**(9):103372

[10] Kannan SR, Spratt AN, Cohen AR, Naqvi SH, Chand HS, Quinn TP, et al. Evolutionary analysis of the delta and delta plus variants of the SARS-CoV-2 viruses. Journal of Autoimmunity. 2021;**124**:102715

[11] Burki TK. Omicron variant and booster COVID-19 vaccines. The Lancet Respiratory Medicine. 2022;**10**(2):e17

[12] Madhi SA, Kwatra G, Myers JE, Jassat W, Dhar N, Mukendi CK, et al. Population immunity and covid-19 severity with omicron variant in South Africa. The New England Journal of Medicine. 2022;**386**(14):1314-1326

[13] Graña C, Ghosn L, Evrenoglou T, Jarde A, Minozzi S, Bergman H, et al. Efficacy and safety of covid-19 vaccines. Cochrane Database of Systematic Reviews. 2022;**12**(12):Cd015477

[14] Groff D, Sun A, Ssentongo AE, Ba DM, Parsons N, Poudel GR, et al. Short-term and long-term rates of

postacute sequelae of SARS-CoV-2 infection: A systematic review. JAMA Network Open. 2021;**4**(10):e2128568

[15] Barbari A. COVID-19 vaccine concerns: Fact or fiction? Experimental and Clinical Transplantation. 2021;**19**(7):627-634

[16] Li Z, Tao B, Hu Z, Yi Y, Wang J. Effects of short-term ambient particulate matter exposure on the risk of severe COVID-19. The Journal of Infection. 2022;**84**(5):684-691

[17] Zimmermann P, Pittet LF, Finn A, Pollard AJ, Curtis N. Should children be vaccinated against COVID-19? Archives of Disease in Childhood. 2022;**107**(3):e1

[18] Martín Sánchez FJ, Martínez-Sellés M, Molero García JM, Moreno Guillén S, Rodríguez-Artalejo FJ, Ruiz-Galiana J, et al. Insights for COVID-19 in 2023. Revista Española de Quimioterapia. 2023;**36**(2):114-124

[19] Zhang HP, Sun YL, Wang YF, Yazici D, Azkur D, Ogulur I, et al. Recent developments in the immunopathology of COVID-19. Allergy. 2023;**78**(2):369-388

[20] Niemi MEK, Daly MJ, Ganna A. The human genetic epidemiology of COVID-19. Nature Reviews. Genetics. 2022;**23**(9):533-546

[21] Ghram A, Ayadi H, Knechtle B, Ben SH. What should a family physician know about nutrition and physical exercise rehabilitation' advices to communicate to 'long-term COVID-19′ patients? Postgraduate Medicine. 2022;**134**(2):143-147

[22] Aitken Z, Emerson E, Kavanagh AM. COVID-19 vaccination coverage and vaccine hesitancy among Australians with disability and long-term health conditions. Health Promotion Journal of Australia. Oct 2023;**34**(4):895-902. DOI: 10.1002/hpja.691. Epub 2023 Jan 11. PMID: 36565293; PMCID: PMC9880664

[23] Petersen E, Gökengin D, Al Balushi A, Zumla A. One and a half years into the COVID-19 pandemic - exit strategies and efficacy of SARS-CoV-2 vaccines for holistic management and achieving global control. Turkish Journal of Medical Sciences. 2021;**51**(Si-1):3157-3161

[24] Ghersi D, Pang T. En route to international clinical trial transparency. Lancet. 2008;**372**(9649):1531-1532

[25] World Health Organization. International Standards for Clinical Trial Registries: The Registration of all Interventional Trials Is a Scientific, Ethical and Moral Responsibility. version 3.0 ed. Geneva: World Health Organization; 2018

[26] Ndwandwe DE, Runeyi S, Pienaar E, Mathebula L, Hohlfeld A, Wiysonge CS. Practices and trends in clinical trial registration in the pan African clinical trials registry (PACTR): A descriptive analysis of registration data. BMJ Open. 2022;**12**(1):e057474

[27] World Health Organization. International Clinical Trials Registry Platform (ICTRP). World Health Organization. Available from: https://www.who.int/clinical-trials-registry-platform; [Accessed: August 3, 2023]

[28] Holshue ML, DeBolt C, Lindquist S, Lofy KH, Wiesman J, Bruce H, et al. First case of 2019 novel coronavirus in the United States. The New England Journal of Medicine. 2020;**382**(10):929-936

[29] Mallapaty S. Where did omicron come from? Three key theories. Nature. 2022;**602**(7895):26-28

[30] Alu A, Chen L, Lei H, Wei Y, Tian X, Wei X. Intranasal COVID-19 vaccines: From bench to bed. eBioMedicine. 2022;**76**:103841

[31] Huang X, Biswas S, Oki Y, Issa JP, Berry DA. A parallel phase I/II clinical trial design for combination therapies. Biometrics. 2007;**63**(2):429-436

[32] Vilches TN, Nourbakhsh S, Zhang K, Juden-Kelly L, Cipriano LE, Langley JM, et al. Multifaceted strategies for the control of COVID-19 outbreaks in long-term care facilities in Ontario, Canada. Preventive Medicine. 2021;**148**:106564

[33] Williams J, Degeling C, McVernon J, Dawson A. How should we conduct pandemic vaccination? Vaccine. 2021;**39**(6):994-999

[34] Güner R, Hasanoğlu I, Aktaş F. COVID-19: Prevention and control measures in community. Turkish Journal of Medical Sciences. 2020;**50**(Si-1):571-577

[35] Dzinamarira T, Murewanhema G, Musuka G. Different SARS-CoV-2 variants, same prevention strategies. Public Health Practice (Oxf). 2022;**3**:100223

[36] Lam HY, Lau CCA, Wong CH, Lee KYK, Yip SL, Tsang KLA, et al. A review of epidemiology and public health control measures of COVID-19 variants in Hong Kong, December 2020 to June 2021. IJID Regions. 2022;**2**:16-24

[37] Dai L, Gao GF. Viral targets for vaccines against COVID-19. Nature Reviews. Immunology. 2021;**21**(2):73-82

[38] COVID-19 Forecasting Team. Past SARS-CoV-2 infection protection against re-infection: A systematic review and meta-analysis. Lancet. 11 Mar 2023;**401**(10379):833-842. DOI: 10.1016/S0140-6736(22)02465-5. Epub 2023 Feb 16. PMID: 36930674; PMCID: PMC9998097

[39] Gęca T, Wojtowicz K, Guzik P, Góra T. Increased risk of COVID-19 in patients with diabetes mellitus-current challenges in pathophysiology, treatment and prevention. International Journal of Environmental Research and Public Health. 2022;**19**(11):6555

[40] Vitiello A, Ferrara F. Brief review of the mRNA vaccines COVID-19. Inflammopharmacology. 2021;**29**(3):645-649

[41] Chen CWS, So MKP, Liu FC. Assessing government policies' impact on the COVID-19 pandemic and elderly deaths in East Asia. Epidemiology and Infection. 2022;**150**:e161

[42] Farhangnia P, Dehrouyeh S, Safdarian AR, Farahani SV, Gorgani M, Rezaei N, et al. Recent advances in passive immunotherapies for COVID-19: The evidence-based approaches and clinical trials. International Immunopharmacology. 2022;**109**:108786

[43] Dyer AH, Fallon A, Noonan C, Dolphin H, O'Farrelly C, Bourke NM, et al. Managing the impact of COVID-19 in nursing homes and long-term care facilities: An update. Journal of the American Medical Directors Association. 2022;**23**(9):1590-1602

[44] Fosdick BK, Bayham J, Dilliott J, Ebel GD, Ehrhart N. Model-based evaluation of policy impacts and the continued COVID-19 risk at long term care facilities. Infectious Disease Modelling. 2022;**7**(3):463-472

[45] Schwarz M, Mzoughi S, Lozano-Ojalvo D, Tan AT, Bertoletti A, Guccione E. T cell immunity is key to the pandemic endgame: How to measure and monitor it. Current Research in Immunology. 2022;**3**:215-221

Chapter 11

Impact of New COVID-19 Variant on Stroke, Thrombosis and Neurological Impairment

Richa Das, Shreni Agrawal, Nancy Singh, Kajal Singh and Amit Kumar Tripathi

Abstract

Severe acute respiratory syndrome coronavirus 2 (SARS-CoV-2) infection has devastated the world with coronavirus disease 2019 (COVID-19). SARS-CoV-2 is an RNA virus that has a high mutation rate producing a new variant with serious threats. Recently emerged delta variant (B.1.617.2) (India), and omicron (B.1.1.529) (South Africa) mutant makes more serious attention than others previously known. These variants exhibit many neurological complications. The new variants of COVID-19 are also involved in gut microbiota dysbiosis, thus enhancing inflammation process which in then causes stroke, diabetes and thrombosis. Administering vaccines is crucial due to continual mutation and the introduction of variants of concern. Therefore, variant modified vaccines have been thought of as potential vaccines.

Keywords: COVID-19, gut microbiota dysbiosis, stroke, thrombosis, neurological complication

1. Introduction

In December 2019 an outbreak of pneumonia and respiratory problems occurred in Wuhan city of China making it a complete lockdown within months. The virus which was associated with the outbreak was corona virus disease 2019 (COVID-19). The coronavirus disease is brought on by the enveloped, positive sense single stranded genome virus (++sRNA) known as SARS-CoV-2 (formerly known as 2019-nCoV). The symptoms consist of respiratory distress, fever, cough, fatigue and overall low immunity [1]. Thousands of people died all over the world and in 2020 WHO declared it as worldwide pandemic. SARS-CoV-2 virus was first identified by Tyrell and Bynoe in 1965 from the patients having common cold [2]. SARS CoV-2 has been rapidly evolving, leading to emergence of new strain which fostered the need of new and more adaptive diagnostic methods to tackle the strain. Every other strain showcases different range of symptoms within infected people [2]. SARS-CoV-2 detection methods mostly focus on anti-SARS-CoV-2 antibodies (serological testing), antigen specific viral protein or particular viral nucleic acid (molecular testing). Administering vaccines is crucial due to SARS-CoV-2's continual mutation and the

IntechOpen

introduction of variants of concern. The majority of SARS-CoV-2 vaccines now on market are inactivated, live attenuated, viral vector, protein subunit, RNA and DNA vaccines. Comirnaty, spikevox and vaxveria, the precursor COVID-19 vaccines, received Emergency Use Authorization (EUA) in December 2020, less than a year after the epidemic. There were 40 vated EUA worldwide as of August 2022, with over 11 billion doses administered [3]. Despite this amazing accomplishments, fresh issues have emerged that pose a threat to the pandemics long term control. These issues include newly emerging viral variants with higher transmissibility and immune escape, waning immunity over time in those who have received vaccinations and uncommon but potentially serious vaccines associated adverse events. In this book chapter, we will cover the molecular mechanism of COVID-19 new variants, impact on gut microbiota and neurological complications. We will also discuss the bivalent, nasal and oral Vaccines against COVID-19, along with the variant modified COVID-19 vaccines.

2. Molecular mechanism of action of COVID-19 new variant

SARS-CoV-2 uses the S protein to attach to the host cell surface receptor ACE2 (angiotensin-converting enzyme 2) and enters the cell by membrane fusion using type II transmembrane serine protease (TMPRSS2) or cathepsin L and Furin [4]. The S protein is composed of S1 and S2 subunits [5]. The S1 subunit has the RBD (receptor-binding domain), which binds to ACE2. The S2 subunit has the transmembrane part of the S protein, which anchors the S protein to the membrane and helps the viral and cellular membranes fuse together [6, 7]. Several investigations have demonstrated that Omicron RBD binds ACE2 1.5–2.8 times better than the wild-type [8]. Cleavage of the S protein at the S1–S2 and S2 sites is required for virus to enter host cell. Cathepsin L and Furin are responsible for carrying this out. TMPRSS2 and cathepsin L can cleave the SARS-CoV-2 genome at the S2 location, which results in two distinct entry points for the virus into cells. Because it is located on the exterior of the cell, TMPRSS2 regulates the passage of substances via plasma membrane. The process of entering the endosome is regulated by cathepsin L, which is located within the endosome. [6, 9–11] Six distinct mutations on S2 (N764K, D796Y, N856K, Q954H, N969K, and L981F) are present in the Omicron variation and have not been found in prior VOCs [12]. Recent research has shown that the Omicron spike pseudo typed virus prefers endosomal entrance over plasma membrane entry, and that infection was decreased in TMPRSS2 expressing cells but enhanced in cells which promote endosomal entry [13–15]. The Omicron variant contains three mutations in the furin cleavage site region (P681H, H655Y, and N679K). Basic mutation P681H in the polybasic cleavage site (PBCS), which is also found in Alpha and Gamma, has been shown to speed up furin-mediated cleavage of the S protein, which could make the virus more infectious [16].

3. Recent variants of COVID-19

The World Health Organisation (WHO) reported the Omicron variants as the most recent variant of concern (VOC) that emerged on November 26, 2021. The Omicron variant lineage is divided into the following sub-lineages: BA.1 (B.1.1.529

and BA.1.1), BA.2, BA.3, BA.4, and BA.5 [17]. The SARS-CoV-2 spike protein of omicron variant showed total 37 amino acid mutations, a few of which were found in the RBD [18]. The RBD is mostly found in the S protein, which binds to the host receptor angiotensin-converting enzyme 2 (ACE2) and may boost infectivity and facilitate escape from neutralising antibodies brought on by vaccination [19–21]. By February 2022, the first Omicron BA.1 lineage had been replaced by the BA.2 lineage, which has been found in various European and Asian countries [22, 23]. The BA.2 lineage is characterized by 57 mutations, 31 of which are found in the S protein. BA.1 and BA.2 share 12 RBD mutations, including G339D, S373P, S375F, K417N, N440K, S477N, T478K, E484A, Q493R, Q498R, N501Y, and Y505H in which BA.2 has two distinct mutations, S371F and R408S and shares T376A and D405N with BA.3 [24]. Although the BA.2 lineage continues to develop, giving rise to new subvariants as BA.2.12.1, BA.2.75, BA.4, and BA.5. In particular, the BA.4/5 and BA.2.75 subvariants have sparked further diversification of the circulating SARS-CoV-2, leading to the formation of a number of new subvariants, including the BA.4.6, BF.7, BQ.1, and BQ.1.1 (derived from BA.4/5), as well as BA.2.75.2 [25]. In contrast to BA.2.75, the BA.2.75.2 subvariant develops R346T, F486S, and D1199N mutations, notably those on RBD, which have raised concerns about additional immune escape [26]. One study also claimed that the F486S mutation substantially drives the enhanced neutralisation resistance of BA.2.75.2 [25]. In addition, BA.5 has taken over as the predominant subvariant in several countries. It should be noted that the successors of BA.5, such as BQ.1, BQ.1.1, and BF.7, are becoming more prevalent in more than 65 various countries, including China, India, Brazil, and the USA. By 19 November 2022, BQ.1, BQ.1.1, and BF.7 were responsible for 25.5%, 24.2%, and 7.8% of all cases in the United States, respectively [27, 28]. In the whole genome of the BF.7 subvariant of Omicron, 55 mutations have been found in which 32 mutations found in S-protein encoding gene. Furthermore, the BQ.1 and BQ.1.1 variant of omicron was also grown by N460K and K444T mutations which increase its neutralisation resistance to antibodies. In addition to the other mutations in the S-protein, the BQ.1.1 and BF.7 subvariant has a fundamental mutation in a crucial location, such as R346T. This mutation was associated with a greater capacity of the virus to evade neutralising antibodies (nAbs) brought on by prior infection or vaccination [26, 29]. A recent study showed that, compared to the original coronavirus, the BF.7 variant demonstrated 4.4 times greater resistance to neutralisation [25]. When compared with D614G, the BA.4.6, BF.7, BQ.1, and BQ.1.1 subvariants exhibited a 10.6-fold ($p < 0.0001$), 11.0-fold ($p < 0.0001$), 18.7- fold ($p < 0.0001$), and 22.9-fold ($p < 0.0001$) higher neutralization resistance, respectively [25].

4. Impact of COVID-19 on gut microbiota

The gut microbiota is the variety of bacteria that populate the gastrointestinal (GI) tract as part of a complex and dynamic ecosystem [30, 31]. The term eubiosis refers to the balance of different genus or species of bacteria that belongs to the 4 phyla which includes, *Actinobacteria, Proteobacteria, Firmicutes* and *Bacteroidetes* [32]. Any alteration in the composition of the gut microbiota or abnormalities with the gut microbiota's homeostasis is given the term dysbiosis [33]. Numerous studies have documented gut dysbiosis in patients suffering from COVID-19 [34, 35]. Patients with SARS-CoV2 infection have dysbiosis in their gut microbiome, which causes an increase in GI opportunistic bacteria, suggesting a potential connection between SARS-CoV2 and gut-lung axis [36, 37]. The gut microbiome dysbiosis reduces the beneficial commensals that are anti-inflammatory, like, *Lachnospiraceae, Faecalibacterium prausnitzii and Roseburia*, *Eubacterium*, and enriches the gut of the COVID-19 patients with opportunistic pathogens that cause bacteremia such as, *Bacteroides nordii*, *Clostridium hathewayi*, *Actinomyces viscosus* and *Enterobacteriaceae*, *Enterococcus* [38]. Important epithelial cells are altered by the gut microbiome dysbiosis, as seen in K18-hACE2 mice in a study. The ileum of infected mice had significantly more mucus-producing goblet cells and fewer Paneth cells. A decrease in the number of Paneth cells was accompanied by abnormalities, like, misplaced or deformed granules, reduction in the expression of antimicrobial factors like, serum amyloid A, lysozyme, Reg3γ and defensins. This resulted from the sharp variations in Akkermansiaceae concentration [39]. Patients with COVID-19 also showed a depletion of bacteria that produce SCFAs (short-chain fatty acid), such as Parabacteroides, Bacteroides, and Lachnospiraeae. In the presence of SARS-CoV-2, metabolomic studies of animal models observed alterations in SCFA synthesis, which decreased lung defenses, strengthened pathogen colonization and the development of bacterial infection [40–42].

5. Impact of new variant of COVID-19 on neurological complications

Research is ongoing on the clinical importance of SARS-CoV-2 brain infection. It has been discovered that brain infection and inflammation are linked to neurological symptoms in COVID-19 patients, including headache, dizziness, myalgia, disorientation, delirium, and altered mental status [43, 44]. The introduction of the delta (B1.617.2) mutation increased the probability of COVID-19 neurological diagnoses (such as cognitive disability, epilepsy or seizures, and ischemic strokes) [45]. The SARS-CoV-2 delta variant is more virulent than the early strain (Hu-1 variants) and causes severe neurotropic patterns. Histopathological examination of the brains of K18-hACE2 mice showed that B1.617.2 infects the brains more quickly and effectively than Hu-1. It was found that the early activation of several signature genes in delta-infected mice involves innate cytokines, and the necrosis-related response was more prominent than in Hu-1-infected mice [46]. The Omicron variety has currently taken over as the dominant strain, which has led to a pattern of development into the enduring and endemic COVID-19 [47]. Notably, despite the fact that the initial strain led to fatal brain infections in COVID-19 mice models, [48, 49] both adult human cases and animal models infected with Omicron allegedly did not exhibit these symptoms. However, because everyone's immune status varies, the severity of SARS-CoV-2 variations is complex, therefore it's important not to underestimate the pathogenicity brought on by the Omicron variant [50]. Recently, a neonate with the Omicron BA.1 mutation was discovered to have severe encephalopathy [51]. In another recent work, scientists employed K18-hACE mice to show that the Omicron version can infect the brain. Their findings demonstrated that abnormalities in lymphoid organs coexist with Omicron infection in the brain [50]. In comparison to earlier versions, the Omicron variant is also linked to seizures and decreased mental status in youngsters [52].

6. COVID-19, stroke and thrombosis

Based on clinical observation and initial case series, the COVID-19 pandemic is associated with stroke induced neurological impairment [53]. These reported neurological impairments were the anosmia, ageusia, cerebral haemorrhage and infarction [54]. The potential mechanism of ischemic stroke in the older age COVID-19 patients with various comorbidities and severe illness were observed. The uncommon reasons of stroke in the COVID-19 patients are atherosclerosis, hypertension and arterial fibrillation. SARS-CoV-2 virus binds to the angiotensin convertin enzyme-2 (ACE2) present on brain endothelial cells and smooth muscles cells [55, 56]. ACE2 is the key part of the renin angiotensin system (RAS) and the counter balance to the ACE1 and angiotensin II. Angiotensin II is proinflammatory, vasoconstrictive and promotes organ damage. Depletion of ACE2 by the SARS-CoV-2 may tip the balance in the favour of harmful ACE1/angiotensin II axis and promote tissue injury including stroke. Treatment with tissue plasminogen activator for COVID-19 related stroke and low molecular weight of heparinoids may reduce the thrombosis and mortality in sepsis-induced coagulopathy [57]. The three mechanistic pathways involved in the incidence of stroke are hypercoagulable state, vasculitis, and cardiomyopathy. The venous thrombosis has been reported in the patients with severe COVID-19 [58]. However, pathogenesis of hemorrhagic stroke in COVID-19 has not been fully elucidated. It has been postulated that affinity of SARS-CoV-2 for the ACE2 receptors, which are expressed in endothelial and arterial smooth muscles cells in the brain allow the virus to mechanical damage the intra-arterial arteries causing vessel wall rupture [55]. The COVID-19 patients, who had stroke were more likely to be older and have hypertension, diabetes, cancer and higher level of D-dimer [59]. The diagnostic investigations could not be completed in some COVID-19 patients, might have contributed to the high rate of cryptogenic strokes. The cytokine may also damage and result in blood brain barrier (BBB) leakage and cause hemorrhagic posterior reversible encephalopathy syndrome. Several nutritional components such as vitamin D and phytochemicals such as riboflavin and piperine can be essential nutraceutical components may involve in protection and prevention from the ischemic stroke injury (**Figure 1**) [60–62].

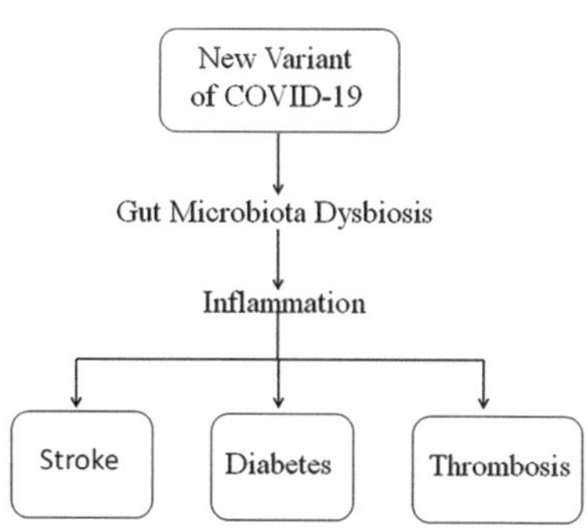

Figure 1.
Impact of new COVID-19 variant on gut microbiota which enhances the inflammation process in various metabolic disease as well as thrombosis.

7. Bivalent, nasal and oral vaccines against COVID-19

A recent report from the World Health Organization (WHO) revealed that seven vaccines (Covishield, Janssen/Ad26, Moderna COVID-19, Sinopharm, Sinovac-CoronaVac, Pfizer/BioNtech, and COVAXIN) have been approved for use against SARS-CoV2 in humans. Most of these immunisations are given as intramuscular injections [63–68]. However, it's crucial to remember that the intramuscular vaccinations only cause a systemic immune response; they have no effect on the mucous membranes. For SARS-CoV2 to be successfully neutralised in the upper respiratory system, mucosal immunity is essential. It aids in preventing the virus's transmission to the lower respiratory system and the development of serious disease. The probability of SARS-CoV2 transmission from immunised persons who might still get the virus and disseminate it increases in the absence of mucosal protection, which entails the generation of local secretory immunoglobulin A (sIgA) antibodies [69]. Fortunately, there has been significant progress in developing mucosal vaccines that can be administered orally or intranasally. These vaccines offer a non-invasive delivery method and can generate mucosal immunity, in addition to humoral and cellular immunity, effectively providing protection against COVID-19 [70, 71]. Vaccines administered orally or intravenously can produce a significant B and T cell–mediated immune response in addition to the intended mucosal protection. A specific study focused on improving the mucosal vaccination for Omicron variants and developed ChAd-SARS-CoV-2-BA.5-S. This vaccine was evaluated in both monovalent and bivalent forms for its efficacy against circulating variations, including BQ.1.1 and XBB.1.5, and produces a pre-fusion and surface-stabilized S protein of the BA.5 strain. According to the study, these vaccinations did not protect against the antigenically distant XBB.1.5 Omicron strain in passive transfer tests because the serum neutralising antibody responses they produced were insufficient. The study did, however, show encouraging outcomes for nasally administered bivalent ChAd-vectored vaccinations. These vaccinations offered immunity to WA1/2020 D614G and Omicron variants BQ.1.1 and XBB.1.5 in both the upper and lower respiratory tracts by inducing strong antibody and spike-specific memory T cell responses in the respiratory mucosa [72].

8. Variant modified COVID-19 vaccines

The COVID-19 vaccine offers significant protection against both symptomatic and severe disease. However, the efficacy of existing vaccination regimens, which are based on the ancestor (Wuhan-like) variant, has been significantly decreased by the introduction of antigenically unique SARS-CoV-2 variants [73]. Current vaccines, such as those based on nucleic acids, viral vectors, subunit vaccines, and inactivated vaccines, were developed based on the generation of potent immune responses against the spike (S) protein of SARS-CoV-2 [74]. The increase in SARS-CoV-2 variants with novel mutations, especially those with appealing mutations collectively referred to as variants of concern (VOCs), have been thought of as potential spike proteins for antigen-based vaccines. The primary causes of immunological escape, resistance to neutralising antibodies, and low efficiency of existing vaccines to prevent infection are the subsequent appearance of SARS-CoV-2 variants bearing novel mutations in the receptor binding domain (RBD) of spike protein [75]. A new phase of the SARS-CoV-2 pandemic may result from Omicron sub-lineages easily recombining and fusing with one another, according to recent findings. As a result, developing a multivalent vaccination can be a successful strategy for combating the new SARSCoV-2 variants, which predominantly emerged as a result of recombination between hybrid forms. In order to offer a greater range of protection against new SARS-CoV-2 variants, the Moderna firm recently created new multivalent vaccines, such as mRNA-1273.351 (targeting the B.1.351) and mRNA-1273.351 (targeting the B.1.351) [76]. Due to having a considerably larger fraction possessing important all RBD epitopes, being much easier to make, having lower production costs, and being more immunogenic, multivalent vaccines may be able to provide stronger immune protection against novel SARS-CoV-2 variants [77]. According to a recent study, multivalent S2-based vaccinations offer extensive protection against VOCs. It was shown that vaccination with S2-based constructs produced an IgG antibody response that was broadly cross-reactive and recognized the spike proteins of VOCs. Importantly, vaccination decreased the viral titers in respiratory tissues of animals exposed to SARS-CoV-2 variants B.1.351 (beta), B.1.617.2 (delta), and BA.1 (omicron) [78]. The current intramuscular COVID-19 vaccinations are at risk of losing their effectiveness due to the emergence of SARS-CoV-2 VOCs. Researchers tested trivalent COVID-19 vaccines expressing spike-1, nucleocapsid, and RdRp antigens in mice models using adenoviral vectors (Ad) of human and chimpanzee origin. They demonstrated that intranasal immunisation, particularly with chimpanzee Ad-vectored vaccine, induces a tripartite protective immunity consisting of local and systemic antibody responses, mucosal tissue-resident memory T cells, and mucosal trained innate immunity, which is superior to intramuscular immunisation. Such intranasal immunisation offers defence against the two VOC, B.1.1.7 and B.1.351, as well as the ancestor SARS-CoV-2. According to their research, an efficient next-generation COVID-19 vaccination method to generate overall mucosal immunity against existing and future VOC is respiratory mucosal administration of the Ad-vectored multivalent vaccine [79, 80].

9. Conclusion and future direction of therapy

The Omicron variant has garnered global attention due to its numerous mutations. There are significant concerns regarding other VoCs, such as Alpha (B.1.1.7), Beta (B.1.351), Gamma (B.1.1.28.1), and Delta (B.1.617.2), as they are associated with higher infectivity, transmission rates, and potential immune evasion mechanisms. A substantial percentage of COVID-19-infected patients, around 15–20%, experience a severe form of acute infection, characterized by hyperinflammatory cytokine storms, resulting in more morbidity and mortality than the actual cytotoxicity of the virus. Furthermore, recent findings suggest the correlation between microbial gut dysbiosis and the severity of the COVID-19 sickness. This has prompted researchers to investigate possible preventative and therapeutic targets including probiotics and dietary changes. Although clinical data suggests that immunopathogenesis, neuroinvasion, neuroinflammation, hypoxia, and neuroinflammation are all involved in the emergence of CNS symptoms, the precise molecular mechanism of COVID-19 neurotoxicity is still not fully characterised. Additionally, a hypercoagulable condition brought on by COVID-19 infection seems to be associated with an increased risk of thrombosis, including cases of ischemic stroke from large-vessel blockage. Given the catastrophic effects of COVID-19 on human lives, the WHO has sped up vaccine development to guarantee that people everywhere may obtain high-quality, safe, and effective vaccinations against SARS-CoV2. According to a recent study, mucosal vaccinations given intranasally after the first intramuscular vaccination may operate as booster doses, triggering a strong immune response that aids in preventing the reproduction of SARS-CoV2 in the upper and lower respiratory tracts. Future examination of the vaccines now under development, including the assessment of extensive clinical investigations and trials, may pave the way for the availability of prospective mucosal vaccines and associated medicines. This can result in their inclusion in international immunisation campaigns.

Abbreviations

COVID-19	coronavirus disease of 2019
SARS-CoV-2	severe acute respiratory syndrome coronavirus 2
WHO	World Health Organization
ACE2	angiotensin-converting enzyme 2
TMPRSS2	transmembrane serine protease 2
PBCS	polybasic cleavage site
RBD	receptor-binding domain
VOC	variant of concern
nAbs	neutralising antibodies
GI	gastrointestinal (GI) tract
SCFA	short-chain fatty acids

Author details

Richa Das[1], Shreni Agrawal[1], Nancy Singh[2], Kajal Singh[2] and Amit Kumar Tripathi[2*]

1 Department of Biotechnology, Parul Institute of Applied Science, Parul University, Vadodara, Gujarat, India

2 Department of Biosciences, Galgotias University, Gautam Buddh Nagar, UP, India

*Address all correspondence to: amitibt2008@gmail.com

References

[1] Rotondo JC, Martini F, Maritati M, Caselli E, Gallenga CE, Guarino M, et al. Advanced molecular and immunological diagnostic methods to detect SARS-CoV-2 infection. Microorganisms. 2022;**10**(6):1193

[2] Tyrrell DAJ, Bynoe ML. Cultivation of a novel type of common-cold virus in organ cultures. British Medical Journal. 1965;**1**:1467-1470. DOI: 10.1136/bmj.1.5448.1467

[3] Li M, Wang H, Tian L, Pang Z, Yang Q, Huang T, et al. COVID-19 vaccine development: Milestones, lessons and prospects. Signal Transduction and Targeted Therapy. 2022;**7**(1):146. DOI: 10.1038/s41392-022-00996-y

[4] Dong Y, Dai T, Liu J, Zhang L, Zhou F. Coronavirus in continuous flux: From SARS-CoV to SARS-CoV-2. Advanced Science (Weinh). 2020;7(20):2001474. DOI: 10.1002/advs.202001474

[5] Wrapp D et al. Cryo-EM structure of the 2019-nCoV spike in the prefusion conformation. Science. 2020;**367**:1260-1263. DOI: 10.1126/science.abb2507

[6] Jackson CB, Farzan M, Chen B, Choe H. Mechanisms of SARS-CoV-2 entry into cells. Nature Reviews Molecular Cell Biology. 2022;**23**:3-20. DOI: 10.1038/s41580-021-00418-x

[7] Bayati A, Kumar R, Francis V, McPherson PS. SARS-CoV-2 infects cells after viral entry via clathrin-mediated endocytosis. The Journal of Biological Chemistry. 2021;**296**:100306

[8] Fan Y, Li X, Zhang L, Wan S, Zhang L, Zhou F. SARS-CoV-2 Omicron variant: Recent progress and future perspectives. Signal Transduction and Targeted Therapy. 2022;7(1):141. DOI: 10.1038/s41392-022-00997x [Accessed: April 28, 2022]

[9] Zhang L, Mann M, Syed ZA, Reynolds HM, Tian E, Samara NL, et al. Furin cleavage of the SARS-CoV-2 spike is modulated by O-glycosylation. Proceedings of the National Academy of Sciences of the United States of America. 2021;**118**(47):e2109905118. DOI: 10.1073/pnas.2109905118

[10] Hoffmann M et al. SARS-CoV-2 cell entry depends on ACE2 and TMPRSS2 and is blocked by a clinically proven protease inhibitor. Cell. 2020;**181**:271-280

[11] Simmons G et al. Inhibitors of cathepsin L prevent severe acute respiratory syndrome coronavirus entry. Proceedings of the National Academy of Sciences of the United States of America. 2005;**102**:11876-11881

[12] Meng B et al. Altered TMPRSS2 usage by SARS-CoV-2 Omicron impacts tropism and fusogenicity. Nature. 2022;**603**:706-714

[13] Rabaan AA, Al-Ahmed SH, Albayat H, Alwarthan S, Alhajri M, Najim MA, et al. Variants of SARS-CoV-2: Influences on the vaccines' effectiveness and possible strategies to overcome their consequences. Medicina. 2023;**59**:507. DOI: 10.3390/medicina59030507

[14] Willett BJ, Grove J, MacLean OA, et al. SARS-CoV-2 Omicron is an immune escape variant with an altered cell entry pathway. Nature Microbiology. 2022;**7**:1161-1179. DOI: 10.1038/s41564-022-01143-7

[15] Zhao H et al. SARS-CoV-2 Omicron variant shows less efficient replication

and fusion activity when compared with Delta variant in TMPRSS2-expressed cells. Emerging Microbes & Infections. 2022;**11**:277-283

[16] Peacock TP et al. The furin cleavage site in the SARS-CoV-2 spike protein is required for transmission in ferrets. Nature Microbiology. 2021;**6**:899-909

[17] Mohseni Afshar Z, Tavakoli Pirzaman A, Karim B, Rahimipour Anaraki S, Hosseinzadeh R, Sanjari Pireivatlou E, et al. SARS-CoV-2 Omicron (B.1.1.529) Variant: A challenge with COVID-19. Diagnostics. 2023;**13**:559

[18] Cameroni E, Bowen JE, Rosen LE, Saliba C, Zepeda SK, Culap K, et al. Broadly neutralizing antibodies overcome SARS-CoV-2 Omicron antigenic shift. Nature. 2022;**602**:664-670

[19] Li Q et al. SARS-CoV-2 501Y. V2 variants lack higher infectivity but do have immune escape. Cell. 2021;**184**:2362-2371. DOI: 10.1016/j.cell.2021.02.042

[20] Garcia-Beltran WF et al. Multiple SARS-CoV-2 variants escape neutralization by vaccine-induced humoral immunity. Cell. 2021;**184**:2372-2383. DOI: 10.1016/j.cell.2021.03.013

[21] Cao Y et al. Humoral immune response to circulating SARS-CoV-2 variants elicited by inactivated and RBD-subunit vaccines. Cell Research. 2021;**31**:732-741. DOI: 10.1038/s41422-021-00514-9

[22] WHO. Weekly Epidemiological Update on COVID-19. 2022. [Accessed: June 9, 2022]

[23] Yamasoba D, Kimura I, Nasser H, Morioka Y, Nao N, Ito J, et al. Virological characteristics of the SARS-CoV-2 Omicron BA.2 spike. Cell. 2022;**185**:2103-2115.e19. DOI: 10.1016/j.cell.2022.04.035

[24] Greaney AJ et al. Complete mapping of mutations to the SARS-CoV-2 spike receptor-binding domain that escape antibody recognition. Cell Host & Microbe. 2021;**29**:44-57. DOI: 10.1016/j.chom.2020.11.007

[25] Qu P, Evans JP, Faraone JN, Zheng YM, Carlin C, Anghelina M, et al. Enhanced neutralization resistance of SARS-CoV-2 Omicron subvariants BQ.1, BQ.1.1, BA.4.6, BF.7, and BA.2.75.2. Cell Host & Microbe. 2023;**31**:9-17.e13

[26] Cao Y, Jian F, Wang J, Yu Y, Song W, Yisimayi A, et al. Imprinted SARS-CoV-2 humoral immunity induces convergent Omicron RBD evolution. Nature. 2023;**614**(7948):521-529. DOI: 10.1038/s41586-022-05644-7

[27] Sagar V. What is BF.7, COVID variant spreading in China & does India need to worry? In: Symptoms, Infection Rate Explained. NEWS18 2022;

[28] World Health Organization. TAG-VE Statement on Omicron Sublineages BQ.1 and XBB. Geneva, Switzerland: World Health Organization; 2022

[29] Chakraborty C, Bhattacharya M, Chopra H, Bhattacharya P, Islam MA, Dhama K. Recently emerged omicron subvariant BF.7 and its R346T mutation in the RBD region reveal increased transmissibility and higher resistance to neutralization antibodies: Need to understand more under the current scenario of rising cases in China and fears of driving a new wave of the COVID-19 pandemic. International Journal of Surgery. 2023;**109**(4):1037-1040. DOI: 10.1097/JS9.0000000000000219

[30] Bäckhed F, Ley RE, Sonnenburg JL, Peterson DA, Gordon JI. Host-bacterial

mutualism in the human intestine. Science. 2005;**307**(5717):1915-1920

[31] Thursby E, Juge N. Introduction to the human gut microbiota. The Biochemical Journal. 2017;**474**(11):1823-1836

[32] SeyedAlinaghi S, Afzalian A, Pashaei Z, Varshochi S, Karimi A, Mojdeganlou H, et al. Gut microbiota and COVID-19: A systematic review. Health Science Reports. 2023;**6**(2):e1080. DOI: 10.1002/hsr2.1080

[33] Lloyd-Price J, Abu-Ali G, Huttenhower C. The healthy human microbiome. Genome Medicine. 2016;**8**(1):51

[34] Das R, Singh R, Tripathi AK. Gut microbiome, COVID-19, and neurological impairment. In: Tripathi AK, Kotak M, editors. Gut Microbiome in Neurological Health and Disorders. Nutritional Neurosciences. Singapore: Springer; 2022. DOI: 10.1007/978-981-19-4530-4_14

[35] Farsi Y, Tahvildari A, Arbabi M, et al. Diagnostic, prognostic, and therapeutic roles of gut microbiota in COVID-19: A comprehensive systematic review. Frontiers in Cellular and Infection Microbiology. 2022;**12**:804644

[36] Han Y, Jia Z, Shi J, Wang W, He K. The active lung microbiota landscape of COVID-19 patients through the metatranscriptome data analysis. BioImpacts: BI. 2022;**12**(2):139-146

[37] Baradaran Ghavami S, Pourhamzeh M, Farmani M, et al. Cross-talk between immune system and microbiota in COVID-19. Expert Review of Gastroenterology & Hepatology. 2021;**15**(11):1281-1294

[38] Zuo T et al. Alterations in gut microbiota of patients with COVID-19 during time of hospitalization. Gastroenterology. 2020;**159**:944-955

[39] Bernard-Raichon L, Venzon M, Klein J, Axelrad JE, Zhang C, Sullivan AP, et al. Gut microbiome dysbiosis in antibiotic-treated COVID-19 patients is associated with microbial translocation and bacteremia. Nature Communications. 2022;**13**(1):5926. DOI: 10.1038/s41467-022-33395-6

[40] Michelle GR, Garrett WS. Gut microbiota, metabolites and host immunity. Nature Reviews. Immunology. 2016;**16**:341-352

[41] Sencio V, Barthelemy A, Tavares LP, Machado MG, Soulard D, Cuinat C, et al. Gut dysbiosis during influenza contributes to pulmonary pneumococcal superinfection through altered short-chain fatty acid production. Cell Reports. 2020;**30**:2934-2947

[42] Sokol H, Contreras V, Maisonnasse P, Desmons A, Delache B, Sencio V, et al. SARS-CoV-2 infection in nonhuman primates alters the composition and functional activity of the gut microbiota. Gut Microbes. 2021;**13**:1-19

[43] Maury A, Lyoubi A, Peiffer-Smadja N, et al. Neurological manifestations associated with SARS-CoV-2 and other coronaviruses: A narrative review for clinicians. Revista de Neurologia. 2021;**177**:51-64. DOI: 10.1016/j.neurol.2020.10.001

[44] Harapan BN, Yoo HJ. Neurological symptoms, manifestations, and complications associated with severe acute respiratory syndrome coronavirus 2 (SARS-CoV-2) and coronavirus disease 19 (COVID-19). Journal of Neurology. 2021;**268**(9):3059-3071. DOI: 10.1007/s00415-021-10406-y

[45] Taquet M, Sillett R, Zhu L, Mendel J, Camplisson I, Dercon Q, et al. Neurological and psychiatric risk trajectories after SARS-CoV-2 infection: An analysis of 2-year retrospective cohort studies including 1 284 437 patients. Lancet Psychiatry. 2022;**9**(10):815-827. DOI: 10.1016/S2215-0366(22)00260-7

[46] Yang JH, Yang MS, Kim DM, et al. Delta (B1.617.2) variant of SARS-CoV-2 induces severe neurotropic patterns in K18-hACE2 mice. Scientific Reports. 2023;**13**:3303. DOI: 10.1038/s41598-023-29909-x

[47] Tiecco G, Storti S, Degli Antoni M, Focà E, Castelli F, Quiros-Roldan E. Omicron genetic and clinical peculiarities that may overturn SARS-CoV-2 pandemic: A literature review. International Journal of Molecular Sciences. 2022;**23**(4):1987. DOI: 10.3390/ijms23041987

[48] Seehusen F, Clark JJ, Sharma P, Bentley EG, Kirby A, Subramaniam K, et al. Neuroinvasion and neurotropism by SARS-CoV-2 variants in the K18-hACE2 mouse. Viruses. 2022;**14**(5):1020. DOI: 10.3390/v14051020

[49] Jeong H, Woo Lee Y, Park IH, Noh H, Kim SH, Kim J, et al. Comparison of the pathogenesis of SARS-CoV-2 infection in K18-hACE2 mouse and Syrian golden hamster models. Disease Models & Mechanisms. 2022;**15**(11):dmm049632. DOI: 10.1242/dmm.049632

[50] Lee NY, Lee YW, Hong SM, On D, Yoon GM, An SH, et al. SARS-CoV-2 Omicron variant causes brain infection with lymphoid depletion in a mouse COVID-19 model. Laboratory Animal Research. 2023;**39**(1):8. DOI: 10.1186/s42826-023-00157-4

[51] Tetsuhara K, Akamine S, Matsubara Y, et al. Severe encephalopathy associated with SARS-CoV-2 Omicron BA.1 variant infection in a neonate. Brain & Development. 2022;**44**:743-747. DOI: 10.1016/j.braindev.2022.06.010

[52] Sahin A, Karadag-Oncel E, Buyuksen O, Ekemen-Keles Y, Ustundag G, Elvan-Tuz A, et al. The diversity in the clinical features of children hospitalized with COVID-19 during the nonvariant, Alpha (B.1.1.7), Delta (B.1.617.2), and Omicron (B.1.1.529) variant periods of SARS CoV-2: Caution for neurological symptoms in Omicron variant. Journal of Medical Virology. 2023;**95**(3):e28628. DOI: 10.1002/jmv.28628

[53] Beyrouti R, Adams ME, Benjamin L, Cohen H, Farmer SF, Goh YY, et al. Characteristics of ischaemic stroke associated with COVID-19. Journal of Neurology, Neurosurgery & Psychiatry. 2020;**91**(8):889-891

[54] Aghagoli G, Gallo Marin B, Katchur NJ, Chaves-Sell F, Asaad WF, Murphy SA. Neurological involvement in COVID-19 and potential mechanisms: A review. Neurocritical Care. 2021;**34**:1062-1071

[55] Carod-Artal FJ. Neurological complications of coronavirus and COVID-19. Revista de Neurologia. 2020;**70**(9):311-322

[56] Singh RS, Singh AK, Shukla KK, Tripathi AK. COVID-19 pandemic: Evidences from clinical studies. Journal of Community and Public Health Nursing. 2020;**6**(4):251

[57] Miesbach W, Makris M. COVID-19: Coagulopathy, risk of thrombosis, and the rationale for anticoagulation. Clinical and Applied Thrombosis/Hemostasis. 2020;**16**:1076029620938149

[58] Loo J, Spittle DA, Newnham M. COVID-19, immunothrombosis and

venous thromboembolism: Biological mechanisms. Thorax. 2021;**76**(4):412-420

[59] Qureshi AI, Abd-Allah F, Al-Senani F, Aytac E, Borhani-Haghighi A, Ciccone A, et al. Management of acute ischemic stroke in patients with COVID-19 infection: Report of an international panel. International Journal of Stroke. 2020;**15**(5):540-554

[60] Tripathi AK, Mishra SK. A review article on neuroprotective, immunomodulatory, and anti-inflammatory role of vitamin-D3 in elderly COVID-19 patients. The Egyptian Journal of Neurology, Psychiatry and Neurosurgery. 2023;**59**(1):1-6

[61] Tripathi AK, Ray AK, Mishra SK, Bishen SM, Mishra H, Khurana A. Molecular and therapeutic insights of alpha-lipoic acid as a potential molecule for disease prevention. Revista Brasileira de Farmacognosia. 2023;**33**(2):272-287

[62] Tripathi AK, Ray AK, Mishra SK. Molecular and pharmacological aspects of piperine as a potential molecule for disease prevention and management: Evidence from clinical trials. Beni-Suef University Journal of Basic and Applied Sciences. 2022;**11**(1):16

[63] Baden LR, El Sahly HM, Essink B, et al. Efficacy and safety of the mRNA-1273 SARS-CoV-2 vaccine. The New England Journal of Medicine. 2020;**384**(5):403-416. DOI: 10.1056/NEJMoa2035389

[64] Logunov DY, Dolzhikova IV, Shcheblyakov DV, et al. Safety and efficacy of an rAd26 and rAd5 vector-based heterologous prime-boost COVID-19 vaccine: An interim analysis of a randomised controlled phase 3 trial in Russia. Lancet. 2021;**397**(10275):671-681. DOI: 10.1016/s0140-6736(21)00234-8

[65] Polack FP, Thomas SJ, Kitchin N, et al. Safety and efficacy of the BNT162b2 mRNA Covid-19 vaccine. The New England Journal of Medicine. 2020;**383**(27):2603-2615. DOI: 10.1056/NEJMoa2034577

[66] Ramasamy MN, Minassian AM, Ewer KJ, et al. Safety and immunogenicity of ChAdOx1 nCoV-19 vaccine administered in a prime-boost regimen in young and old adults (COV002): A single-blind, randomised, controlled, phase 2/3 trial. Lancet. 2021;**396**(10267):1979-1993. DOI: 10.1016/s0140-6736(20)32466-1

[67] Sadoff J, Le Gars M, Shukarev G, et al. Interim results of a phase 1-2a trial of Ad26.COV2.S Covid-19 vaccine. The New England Journal of Medicine. 2021;**384**(19):1824-1835. DOI: 10.1056/NEJMoa2034201

[68] Xia S, Zhang Y, Wang Y, et al. Safety and immunogenicity of an inactivated SARS-CoV-2 vaccine, BBIBP-CorV: A randomised, double-blind, placebo-controlled, phase 1/2 trial. The Lancet Infectious Diseases. 2021;**21**(1):39-51. DOI: 10.1016/s1473-3099(20)30831-8

[69] Russell MW, Moldoveanu Z, Ogra PL, Mestecky J. Mucosal immunity in COVID-19: A neglected but critical aspect of SARS-CoV-2 infection. Perspective. 2020;**11**(3221):611337. DOI: 10.3389/fimmu.2020.611337

[70] Tiboni M, Casettari L, Illum L. Nasal vaccination against SARS-CoV-2: Synergistic or alternative to intramuscular vaccines. International Journal of Pharmaceutics. 2021;**603**:120686. DOI: 10.1016/j.ijpharm.2021.120686

[71] Mudgal R, Nehul S, Tomar S. Prospects for mucosal vaccine: Shutting the door on SARS-CoV-2. Human

Vaccines & Immunotherapeutics. 2020;**16**(12):2921-2931. DOI: 10.1080/21645515.2020.1805992

[72] Ying B, Darling TL, Desai P, Liang CY, Dmitriev IP, Soudani N, et al. A bivalent ChAd nasal vaccine protects against SARS-CoV-2 BQ.1.1 and XBB.1.5 infection and disease in mice and hamsters. bioRxiv [Preprint]. 2023:539332. DOI: 10.1101/2023.05.04.539332

[73] Khoury DS, Docken SS, Subbarao K, et al. Predicting the efficacy of variant-modified COVID-19 vaccine boosters. Nature Medicine. 2023;**29**:574-578. DOI: 10.1038/s41591-023-02228-4

[74] Chiba S, Frey SJ, Halfmann PJ, Kuroda M, Maemura T, Yang JE, et al. Multivalent nanoparticle-based vaccines protect hamsters against SARSCoV-2 after a single immunization. Communications Biology. 2021;**4**(1):1-9

[75] Uttamrao PP, Sathyaseelan C, Patro LP, Rathinavelan T. Revelation of potent epitopes present in unannotated ORF antigens of SARS-CoV-2 for epitope-based polyvalent vaccine design using immunoinformatics approach. Frontiers in Immunology. 2021;**12**:1664-3224

[76] Li T, Huang T, Guo C, Wang A, Shi X, Mo X, et al. Genomic variation, origin tracing, and vaccine development of SARS-CoV-2: A systematic review. The Innovations. 2021;**2**(2):100116

[77] Ghazvini K, Keikha M. Multivalent vaccines against new SARS-CoV-2 hybrid variants. Vacunas. 2023;**24**(1):76-77

[78] Halfmann PJ, Frey SJ, Loeffler K, Kuroda M, Maemura T, Armbrust T, et al. Multivalent S2-based vaccines provide broad protection against SARS-CoV-2 variants of concern and pangolin coronaviruses. eBioMedicine. 2022;**86**:104341. DOI: 10.1016/j.ebiom.2022.104341

[79] Afkhami S, D'Agostino MR, Zhang A, Stacey HD, Marzok A, Kang A, et al. Respiratory mucosal delivery of next-generation COVID-19 vaccine provides robust protection against both ancestral and variant strains of SARS-CoV-2. Cell. 2022;**185**(5):896-915.e19. DOI: 10.1016/j.cell.2022.02.005

[80] Kumar R, Srivastava Y, Muthuramalingam P, Singh SK, Verma G, Tiwari S, et al. Understanding mutations in human SARS-CoV-2 spike glycoprotein: A systematic review & meta-analysis. Viruses. 2023;**15**(4):856. DOI: 10.3390/v15040856